Diabetes

Also by Massachusetts General Hospital

Prostate Disease
Menopause

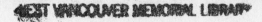
Diabetes

The Most Comprehensive, Up-to-Date Information
Available to Help You Understand Your Condition,
Make the Right Treatment Choices,
and Cope Effectively

David M. Nathan, M.D.
with John F. Lauerman

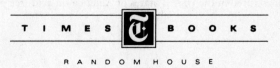

TIMES 𝕿 BOOKS

RANDOM HOUSE

This book cannot and must not replace hands-on medical care or the specific advice of your doctor. Use it instead to help you ask the right questions, make the right choices, and work more closely with your doctor and other members of your health-care team.

To my parents,
who gave me a sense of humor,
and to Ellen, Josh, and Ben,
who have made it only
occasionally necessary
DMN

To Judi,
who made it possible,
and Hanna and James,
who make it worthwhile
JFL

Preface

If you are reading this book, it is likely that you have diabetes mellitus. This is not a lucky guess on my part; diabetes represents possibly the most common chronic disease in the world. Diabetes comes in two "flavors," one of which is relatively rare and tends to develop in childhood or adolescence, and a much more "popular" variety that affects as much as 10 percent of the adult population and usually occurs in older persons. Diabetes is unique among chronic diseases in that it requires a large degree of involvement and effort on the part of the patient. Diabetes affects virtually every aspect of living for those who develop it; it can also have a significant impact on the lives of family members and significant others.

I wrote this book to help you understand the extensive impact that diabetes may have on your life. The more you understand your illness, the better care you'll take of yourself. If this illness affects a family member or other loved one, you will be better prepared to assist in his or her care. Here you will find descriptions of the various forms of diabetes and their causes; discussions of how diabetes may affect aspects of daily living, including exercise and diet; the latest information on the treatment of diabetes; the effects of other diseases on the course and care of diabetes;

the effects of pregnancy; the long-term outcome; and important methods to detect and decrease the complications that can take a serious toll.

The diagnosis and treatment of diabetes have become more sophisticated and increasingly high tech in the past ten years. Not only can doctors diagnose diabetes with improved accuracy and precision, but we increasingly understand its causes and complications, and we have used these insights to improve the care of persons with diabetes. While prevention is not yet a reality, studies toward this end are underway.

The best sources of information about diabetes are often your physician, diabetes educator, dietitian, ophthalmologist, podiatrist, or one of the many other health care professionals who are trained to deal with the day-to-day care of persons with diabetes. But, more so than any other disease, the care of diabetes rests in your hands. In this case, knowledge really is power, the power to control your diabetes and make sure that your day-to-day and long-term quality of life are the best they can be. This book is designed to equip you with that knowledge and that power.

—David M. Nathan, M.D.

Acknowledgments

I owe an unpayable debt of gratitude to my patients who have taught me all of the really important lessons about health, disease, and especially about the human spirit. My colleagues and partners in clinical care and research, Drs. John E. Godine, Joseph Avruch, Lloyd Axelrod, and Enrico Cagliero; clinical and research nurses Kathy Hurxthal, Mary Larkin, Charles McKitrick, and Sue Crowell; dietitians Linda Delahanty and Ellen Anderson; behaviorist Dennis Norman; and a large number of ophthalmologists, podiatrists, surgeons, nephrologists, and others have all contributed to the team effort that characterizes clinical care and research in diabetes at the Mass General. The staff of the Mallinckrodt General Clinical Research Center has been essential in performing many of our studies over the years. Finally, the national and international community of diabetes care providers and investigators, with whom I have been privileged to collaborate, have all contributed in incalculable ways to the advances in science and medicine that continue to improve the lives of people with diabetes.

DMN

I would like to thank everyone from the Massachusetts General Hospital Diabetes Unit, and particularly Dr. David Nathan, Dr. John Godine, Kathy Hurxthal, and Linda Delahanty for their help. I would also like to thank the many other specialists who gave interviews for this book, especially Drs. Hugh Auchincloss, Joseph Avruch, Robert Blatman, Denise Faustman, Lynne Levitsky, Glenn LaMuraglia and Robert Scardina. I would particularly like to thank all the patients who unselfishly offered their time, experiences, and expertise so that this book could be written.

JFL

Contents

Preface   vii

Acknowledgments   ix

Introduction   xiii

1. What Is Diabetes?   3

2. Diagnosis   25

3. The Treatment Team   38

4. Diet: Food for Life   55

5. Insulin: An Owner's Manual   83

6. Exercise: Discover Your Own Fitness
Prescription   114

7. Hypoglycemia   129

8. Complications of Diabetes   145

9. Diabetes and Pregnancy   204

10. Special Considerations for Non-Insulin-
Dependent Diabetes Mellitus (NIDDM)   225

11. The Diabetes Control and Complications
Trial: The New Frontier of Diabetes Care   254

Index   273

Introduction

by John F. Lauerman

I met my wife, Judi, eight years ago at a party in Cambridge, not two miles away from the Massachusetts General Hospital. It was late and we were talking about all the latest films that had recently come out about jazz musicians, and I asked her whether she'd like to go out and see one of them. And, just to make it an evening, I asked her if she'd like to have dinner, too.

The next night, as we sat in a Harvard Square restaurant, looking over the menu and trying to keep our jittery conversation rolling forward, Judi did something that at the time seemed no more than a curiosity, but I now see as brave and, in a way, a crossroads for me as well as her. She took a small black and white padded cosmetic case from the black leather backpack she carried everywhere with her. Inside the case was an unfamiliar apparatus about the size of a paperback book. It looked like a transistor radio.

I had no idea what the device was, and immediately asked, "What's that for?"

"It's my monitor," Judi replied, taking a plastic lancet from the case. She pricked her finger and a small ball of blood welled from her fingertip, which she allowed to drip onto the end of a thin strip of white plastic. "I was diagnosed with type I diabetes two years ago," she added.

I immediately began to worry about whether I knew enough about diabetes to have a conversation about it. After all, I was a medical writer, wasn't I? Shouldn't I know something substantial about one of the most widespread chronic diseases in the United States? Weren't there two types, and one of them caused by a virus? Would she go into a coma if she ate dessert?

As these feelings and thoughts slowly mounted and faded, Judi excused herself from the table so she could inject her insulin privately. But something very important had happened. I had no idea at the time that we would go on to fall in love, to get married, to have children. But Judi had acknowledged her diabetes to me, without broadcasting it, without calling undue attention to it, but simply by being herself and doing what she had to do: monitoring her blood sugar. I look back at that moment as the beginning of my diabetes education.

Diabetes is our constant companion. We think about diabetes when we get up in the morning, each time we cook a meal or go out to eat, as we get ready for a day of work, when we're going out for a walk, when we're planning our vacations, and when we're thinking about making love or just getting ready for bed at night. Diabetes is always there, insisting to be taken care of, and retaliating if ignored.

But despite the pains, frustrations, and fear that go along with diabetes, I found something quite unexpected. Diabetes is a great teacher. It instructs you in the merits of living a healthy life, eating sensibly and in moderation at regular intervals, exercising, paying attention to scrapes, cuts, bruises and infections, consuming alcohol moderately, and refusing to smoke cigarettes or use any form of tobacco. It also teaches you the importance of being honest with yourself, of enlisting the help of family and friends in life's battles without becoming dependent. It teaches the importance of enjoying life, because—as any person with diabetes who suffers from complications can tell you—life can be so much worse.

At this point in our lives, with two children and our home to take care of, diabetes seems almost like a walk in the park. Judi checks her blood sugar and takes her insulin, we stick to a sensible diet, and life goes on. It doesn't seem all that oppressive—somehow, we don't really mind it that much. Don't take this the wrong way: I would go to just about any lengths for a cure for Judi's diabetes. There's nothing I would love more than for her to wake up to a morning that didn't include a blood sugar reading and injection. Although she seldom talks about it, I know that she would love just to stop and have a piece of cheesecake in the middle of the day, without giving it a second thought.

But if all we really wanted was to throw out Judi's syringes and insulin vials and her monitor and stop worrying about blood sugars and diet, well, we could do that. A successful pancreas transplant (see Chapter 8), with luck, could ensure that Judi would never again have to prick her finger or stab a needle into her arm for the sake of diabetes. On the other hand, a pancreas transplant brings with it all kinds of other concerns and complications, including a long hospital stay, and a lifetime of medications to prevent rejection of the transplant.

So, to us at least, the inconveniences of Judi's diabetes management seem relatively easy to bear compared with the potential risks of a transplant. It's obvious enough that there are much harder things than having diabetes. As it is, we have a healthy, satisfying life together, in which Judi and I are obliged to watch our diet and exercise as though our lives depended on it, because hers actually does!

Diabetes highlights the personal responsibility each of us bears for his or her own health. We all know that we ought to eat right and get exercise. We all know that smoking causes heart disease and cancer. We all know that it helps to keep a positive attitude about life, that we should try to avoid letting stressful situations get the better of us. We all know that if we don't do these things, there's a good chance we'll pay for it in the long run.

People with diabetes aren't really any different from other people in these respects. The diabetic walks the same road trod by people without diabetes—it's just that for people with diabetes, the road is narrower. People with diabetes confront hard realities about healthy living earlier than most other people. They quickly find that issues such as mealtimes and calories cannot be left to chance. They cannot afford to skip a medication, whether it be a shot of insulin or oral medication. Self-treatment almost stops being part of the disease and starts being part of life, of realizing who you are.

Sometimes it takes people a while to recognize this responsibility. Carmella Clark is a young woman from Massapequa, Long Island, with a wide, easy smile, dark brown curly hair, and blue eyes. When she was diagnosed with diabetes at the age of ten, her mother immediately began taking responsibility for her disease, giving Carmella all of her shots and taking her blood sugars for her. "I was kind of in denial," an adult Carmella admitted in a conversation at her home in Norwood, a suburb of Boston.

Carmella had moved to Massachusetts when her husband found a job with a local trucking company. While we got to know one another, her daughter, Jessie, already endowed with a thick head of hair like her mother's, played at our feet.

"I used to take two shots a day and test myself sporadically," Carmella said. "So who knows what my blood sugar was doing? I had no idea."

It was really her pregnancy with Jessie that convinced her to get into better control, Carmella admitted. She wanted to do everything possible to make sure her baby was healthy, and she was also worried about her own future with diabetes. Her blood sugars were up and down, and her husband was frustrated with her seeming inability to control them. Carmella decided to start using an insulin pump (see Chapter 5). It would take time to learn, and there would be extra expense, but she accepted the extra effort.

"I just decided it was time to grow up," she said. "I also realized that there are times when you're not taking care of yourself, and you feel fine, but you don't know what's going to happen to you later on down the road. Now I test myself four times a day, and take four shots a day. I was on an insulin pump for a long time, and when we do decide to have another baby, I will go back on the pump."

Over the years, Carmella has gone from a young girl who was in horrible control of her illness—really not in any kind of control at all—to being someone who cares about her blood sugar levels, about her health, and about herself, in a way that she never did before. She has taken charge of her diabetes, and that's changed her life.

"It changes the whole way you feel," says Carmella. "I thought I felt good when I was walking around with high blood sugar. But now, when I look back on it, I used to be a lot more moody, and it was probably because of big swings in my blood sugar which I never realized."

People who learn to treat their diabetes effectively often find that it makes a multidimensional change in their lives. Gradually, they learn to stop resenting having diabetes. Having taken control of their diet, they find that other issues in their lives—frustrations at work, problems with relationships—can be mastered as well. Like a person who's just learned to drive, they find that they enjoy being in control, that although the responsibilities are great, the added burdens bring with them hard-fought freedoms. Small victories loom large, and large victories are so much sweeter than ever before.

Compared with any other period in history, this is the best time for a person to have diabetes. Now, more than ever, there is the opportunity for people with diabetes to have long, healthy, well-adjusted lives while making a minimum of sacrifices. Advances in blood testing technology and new insulins have made it possible for people with diabetes to take better control of their blood sugar. Better focus on the physical *and* psychological problems of diabetics has made it easier for them to cope with their disease and move beyond it to reach other important milestones in their lives. Today, people find that they can do anything—including sports at a high level—with diabetes. As you'll see in Chapter 6, which deals with exercise, there are a number of professional athletes who have diabetes.

Given the fast pace of medical discovery, many people with diabetes have also realized another important fact: those who take care of their disease today will be in a better position to take advantage of tomorrow's medical breakthroughs. And breakthroughs there will be; biomedical laboratories all over the nation and the world are searching furiously for new approaches to treating and, perhaps, curing diabetes. New discoveries in gene therapy will undoubtedly have a huge impact on the lives of the next generation of people with diabetes, if not this one. It demands patience and optimism, but the only road to tomorrow's treatments lies through good, responsible self-treatment today.

Living with and loving someone with diabetes has taught me something very important: that no one, not even someone as close as a spouse, a mother, or a family doctor, can take care of your diabetes for you. I can give Judi a glass of juice when her blood sugar gets low and she's disoriented; I can encourage her to exercise when her sugar's high and she's nauseated and uncomfortable. But she owns the disease, not me, and it's up to her to make the best of it she possibly can. Really, nothing I can do will ever help that.

No doctor, nurse, or dietitian can put you on a program guaranteed to make diabetes a thing of the past. Judi and I know that chances are very good that at some time during our lives, we will have to deal with a serious diabetes-related health issue. As good as the treatment team at Massachusetts General Hospital is, they cannot guarantee that their patients will never have an insulin reaction or suffer from diabetic complications.

What the treatment team can do, and do very well, is talk to people about their diabetes, teach them how to live with it and master it, and give patients the freedom to do the type of work they aspire to do, travel to the countries they long to see, play the sports they love, be with the people they care about the most. That's the hope that any intelligent health care professional has for treating patients. And that's the reason for writing this book.

Diabetes

1

What Is Diabetes?

A Hard Word to Hear

When was the first time you heard the word *diabetes*? Did it happen when someone was telling you, "You have diabetes"? Or was it when someone close to you said, "I just found out I have diabetes"? It's a frightening word, and it frightens a lot of people when they realize what it means. In fact, many people refuse to believe that they have diabetes, even when they're drinking water by the gallon and running to the bathroom every five minutes to urinate—two of the more common symptoms of the disease. One of our residents recently told me that one of his fellow physicians-in-training was feeling run-down and depressed. She discovered independently that she had a blood sugar reading of 350 mg/dl—between three and four times the normal level—and still she refused to believe that she had diabetes! Her reaction was: "I can't have diabetes right now." And yet, if she had seen her own symptoms and that level of blood sugar in any of her patients, she would have made the diagnosis of diabetes immediately.

No one *wants* to have diabetes, any more than anyone wants to lose his hair, get hit by a car, or slip on a banana peel and fall down on the sidewalk. It's just something that happens to you. And there's no "good time" to be diagnosed with diabetes; there are always things you would rather be thinking about or doing than monitoring your blood sugar or taking insulin. But like it or not, more than 600,000 new cases of diabetes are diagnosed each year. This is in men and women of all ages and colors, and at all income levels in this country. If you were recently diagnosed, you can count yourself lucky in at least one way: there are many people with diabetes who don't even know they have it, and their health suffers tremendously as a result of going without treatment. You now have the opportunity to do something about it.

At a certain level, we all know that we're each responsible for our own health. It's when illness occurs—whether it's a mild infection or something serious like a cancer—that we turn some of our problems over to a doctor. Lay people just don't have the expertise to cope with these complicated diseases; we count on doctors and other health care professionals to provide us with medicine, instructions, and support.

Diabetes is different. You must become your own health care provider; there's no doctor who can be there each and every day to interpret readings from your blood sugar monitor and give you shots or oral anti-diabetic agents. Few of us could afford to be followed around by a personal dietitian to pass judgment on each meal. Diabetes is a self-managed, self-treated disease. Doctors, nurse educators, and dietitians can help with advice, but no one can do the real work of treating the disease but you.

Aside from the patients and their caregivers and the researchers who devote their careers to the study and treatment of diabetes, not too many people spend much time thinking about this disease. Almost one half of the people who have diabetes don't even know it themselves. But the fact is that diabetes is extremely common, and has become more and more common over the past fifty years. In Americans over the age of forty, diabetes affects 1 in 15 Caucasians, and from 1 in 10 to 1 in 8 blacks and hispanics. In persons over the age of sixty-five, diabetes affects 1 in 5. Dr. Joseph Avruch, a research diabetologist at Mass General, points out that diabetes has begun affecting races of people who never before even knew of diabetes. For example, the people of many Native American cultures lived on subsistence diets until relatively recently. They ate little food, in comparison with the high-calorie, high-fat diet of a modern American. As these people have assimilated, or been forced to assimilate into American culture, their metabolism has seemed unable to make the change; it appears that they cannot handle the plentiful diet and the obesity that often occurs in modern American life, and they develop diabetes in large numbers. In some Native Americans, such as the Pimas, 50 percent of the adults have diabetes.

This example demonstrates how environmental and cultural conditions interact with diabetes. First of all, the more common form of diabetes, non-insulin-dependent diabetes (NIDDM), occurs more often as people get older. NIDDM usually becomes apparent at about the age of forty-five or fifty, and as people get even older, their vulnerability increases. So, as our society has aged, it has become more diabetes-prone. Also, most people living in the United States have access to vast amounts of fat-rich, calorie-laden food. Our lives are like one long trip to the buffet. The vast majority of diabetes occurs in people whose natural rate of metabolism is insufficient to keep pace with the calories they take in (obesity is a major risk factor for diabetes; see Chapter 4). Other changes in the way we live, work, play, and eat have made diabetes more common. Television keeps people sitting down, when once they might have gone out for a walk or worked in the yard. Fewer people work in jobs that require manual labor. More people are sedentary, especially as they get older. All these changes—the older age, increasing weight, and decreasing physical activity of the U.S. population, and the increasing size of specific ethnic groups at particularly high risk for NIDDM—have made Americans more prone to diabetes.

The sharp rise in diagnoses of diabetes—especially in the form that affects older persons, non-insulin-dependent diabetes—has meant startling statistics in terms of disability and death resulting from complications of diabetes. Diabetes is the leading cause of blindness, kidney disease, and amputations in the United States. Each year, between 15,000 and 40,000 people lose their sight because of diabetes. Ten percent of people with diabetes develop kidney disease, and diabetes is the leading cause of patients having to undergo dialysis. Each year, 54,000 people lose a toe, a foot, or a leg to diabetes. People with diabetes are also at much greater risk for all kinds of cardiovascular disease, including heart attack and stroke. An estimated 15 percent of all health care costs in the United States are associated with the care of diabetes and its complications, amounting to approximately $100 billion per year. This cost includes some 5.7 million days of hospitalization because of diabetes.

Diabetes is no nickel-and-dime disease, that much is

clear. Caring for it demands a lot of money, as much as $4,000 per year for persons with insulin-dependent diabetes, according to some recent estimates. But no matter how much money you spend on diabetes care, it will be worth nothing without self-discipline, concentration, a positive attitude, and above all, honesty. Being honest about your diabetes and about how you feel—with yourself, your doctor, and your family—makes the road to successful treatment much smoother.

"One of the behaviors we see most often among diabetics is concealment," says Carol Wool, M.D., a psychiatrist at Mass General who deals with patients who have difficulty dealing with chronic illness, particularly diabetics. "There's a feeling that nobody must know, especially coworkers. Only the closest family members should know. And most diabetics act this way to avoid pity."

Almost any person who knows about diabetes will tell you that one of the most discouraging aspects of the disease is the feeling of aloneness and isolation, the feeling that no one else can understand what he or she is going through on a daily basis. Good diabetes self-treatment demands that you plan your meals, spend a few minutes a day making important decisions, get regular exercise, and seek preventive medical care on a regular basis. That doesn't sound like much. But when it comes to staying in a business meeting that goes through lunch, having a drink after work, or being the only person at a party who can't eat the hors d'oeuvres, that's when it's hard to say, "I have diabetes," and acknowledge that you're a little bit different from other people. I've heard some of my diabetic patients say, "I'd just like to be normal for one day," as though being "normal" were something that could be achieved just through the secretion of a few pancreatic cells.

It's hard being a good diabetic. Some people will try to cajole you into breaking your diet for the sake of having a little fun, then brand you a spoilsport when you refuse. Others may set high standards for you, and act as though you had asked for a personal trainer. People may blame you, assume that you "ate too many sweets" and caused your own diabetes. You may meet people who are afraid to get into a personal relationship with a person with diabetes. Most of the people you deal with in a given day won't know the first thing about diabetes; that can be trouble if one of those people is assuring you that there's no sugar in something you've just ordered at a restaurant, and it turns out to be laced with corn syrup, molasses, brown sugar, or some other sugary sweetener. Every day can be filled with such conflicts and emotional frustrations. In this book, you'll have the opportunity to hear what some people with diabetes have to say about those frustrations, about their attempts to overcome obstacles, and about what has worked and what hasn't.

With all this confusion surrounding diabetes, you may be surprised to find out that it is one of the world's oldest known diseases. Diabetes was first described in writing in 1500 B.C. The ancient Greeks recognized diabetes and about 1700 years ago even gave us the word *diabetes,* which means "to run water through a siphon," a reference to frequent urination, one of diabetes' first apparent symptoms. (In the 1600s, diabetes was called "the pissing evile.") Several hundred years later, it was discovered that the urine of diabetics tasted sweet (don't you wonder how they found out?), and then someone appended the Greek word *mellitus,* which translates as *honey.* This remains the current terminology for diabetes, so that when your doctor says "diabetes mellitus," it actually means something like "that which runs like water through a siphon and tastes like honey."

Although the observation seems trivial, the finding that diabetics had sugar in their urine revealed the central problem of the disease. *Diabetes is the result of a failure of the body to regulate blood sugar levels adequately.* Not even the discoverers of insulin, the key hormone secreted by the pancreas that plays a significant role in controlling these levels, understood that basic fact, at first. Normally, your body keeps fasting blood sugar within a fairly tight range, between 70 and 115 milligrams of sugar per deciliter of blood (all blood sugar measurements are given in this form: mg/dl). Your body also tightly regulates the increase in blood sugar after meals, and this level seldom exceeds 180 mg/dl, and is usually much lower. Your body needs a fairly steady supply of sugar to keep tissues fed and organs running smoothly—especially the brain, which requires a constant supply of sugar for clear thinking and survival.

Insulin is the major hormone controlling blood sugar levels. Until the discovery of insulin, there was no good way to control blood sugar levels in people who had lost the ability to make their own. People who could still produce some insulin could help themselves with a strictly controlled diet. For children, diabetes was uniformly fatal; 50 percent died within one year of diagnosis, and the rest within two to three years. Nothing was more pathetic than the sight of these emaciated children, their bodies starving for nutrition, and their parents desperately hoping that the next breakthrough in research might yield a cure.

Then in 1922, two researchers from the University of Toronto—Frederick Banting, a young surgeon, and

Charles Best, a fourth-year physiology student—isolated a powerful extract from the pancreas of a dog. First to be treated with the potion was a young boy named Leonard Thompson, who began recovering his color and health within hours of his first dose of the pancreatic extract. Within weeks after that discovery, the news of Thompson's recovery spread quickly around the world. So momentous was the discovery that Banting and Best were showered with accolades and shared the prestigious Nobel Prize for their efforts, along with their coworkers, J. J. R. Macleod and J. B. Collip.

The Toronto research team's discovery helped diabetics in two major ways. First, it gave them insulin, the hormone that allowed them to get some basic control over blood sugar. This was of immediate importance to thousands of children with insulin-dependent diabetes mellitus (IDDM), for whom diabetes had formerly been a death sentence. Second, it gave unprecedented insight into the nature of diabetes: to the extent that blood sugar is under control, diabetes is under control. With their blood sugar levels firmly reined in through the use of diet, exercise, and insulin therapy, diabetics who formerly had a year or two of life to hope for after diagnosis, now began to live for years, sometimes even living out normal life spans.

The discovery of insulin was not like the discovery of antibiotics (which took place in the following decade); insulin did not cure diabetes the way penicillin cleared up an infection. But insulin was extremely effective therapy for what had been a uniformly fatal disease. What insulin allowed people with diabetes to do was to replace their missing hormone and natural blood sugar regulation with a synthetic form of regulation—regulation "by hand," as it were.

Insulin solved the short-term effects of diabetes. But when people with diabetes started living longer, they found that they had traded their old problems for new ones: long-term complications for the eyes, kidneys, nervous system, and cardiovascular system. While insulin therapy prevented the rapid, fatal course of insulin-dependent diabetes, it did not normalize blood sugar levels, and after years of chronic high blood sugar levels, complications developed. Small blood vessels in the back of the eye, the retina, became abnormal, sometimes leading to vision loss. A condition called nephropathy, all too often observed in people with diabetes, resulted in a complete loss of kidney function, forcing many patients either to go on dialysis or seek kidney transplants. Many diabetics also suffered from a malfunction of the nervous system, called neuropathy. Neuropathy caused either a loss of feeling in the feet or sometimes severe shooting pains in the legs and feet. Healing of cuts and bruises often was slower in diabetics with poor circulation and poor blood sugar control. People with diabetes also had higher than average rates of cardiovascular disease—heart attacks and strokes. All in all, with the introduction of insulin therapy, rapid death had been traded in for a host of long-term problems.

What can you do to prevent these complications? Research published in 1993 by physician-scientists here at Mass General and at other hospitals showed that all these complications can be prevented and sometimes even reversed through *tight blood sugar control*.

This was an extremely important experiment, for several reasons. First of all, about 1,400 people with insulin-dependent diabetes participated, and their dedication to the study was extraordinary. As one of the organizers of the study, I was amazed that only eight of the people enrolled dropped out during the ten years of the study, which was known as the Diabetes Control and Complications Trial. This is extremely unusual in any experiment, much less one that demanded that patients structure their lives very tightly, keep detailed notes about their blood sugars and daily activities, adhere to a rigorous schedule of tests, and even get up at 2 A.M. to take blood sugar readings.

For people with diabetes, the payoff was huge. The study demonstrated that intensive therapy which reduced average blood sugar levels to the near-normal range could have truly remarkable results in preventing or delaying complications of diabetes, and in slowing progression if complications had already appeared. When participants kept their blood sugar levels under tight control, the risk of the development of retinopathy was reduced by 76 percent; the progression of retinopathy was slowed by 54 percent; the development of early signs of kidney complications were reduced by 39 percent; development of more severe kidney damage was reduced by 54 percent; and the incidence of diabetic neuropathy was reduced by 60 percent. The effectiveness of intensive therapy was so dramatic that the study was stopped before its scheduled end so that these findings could be announced without delay and other people with diabetes could benefit from this new knowledge.

You may wonder why it took so long for this effective approach to blood sugar control to appear. The answer is that it took us a long time to develop tools and methods that allowed the adjustment of insulin administration to match insulin requirements and to provide effective treatment of diabetes. The first four to five decades of insulin treatment were fraught with ignorance, worry, frustration, and failure. Because there was no method available for patients to monitor blood sugar levels on a regular basis, they were effectively in the dark when they had to choose an insulin dose. Many diabetics overtreated themselves with insulin, leading to "insulin reactions" (see Chapter 7). On the other hand, chronic undertreatment with insulin led to persistently high blood sugar levels, which resulted in the development of diabetic complications. The immediate effect of undertreatment is skyrocketing blood sugar levels, which can cause thirst, excessive urination, dehydration, and even coma. However, the long-term complications are at least as fearsome. (We'll discuss these complications in more detail in Chapter 8.)

The really exciting news for people with diabetes today is that technology has made treatment remarkably better in a number of ways:

• In the early 1980s, glucose (blood sugar) monitors became available that give accurate blood sugar readings on a small drop of blood in one minute or less, providing patients with the necessary information to adjust their insulin doses.

• External insulin pumps that permit the administration of insulin in a pattern that more closely mimics the pancreas's normal insulin delivery have come on the market. Using these devices or carefully tailored injection regimens provides near-normal glucose control.

• Implantable insulin pumps have been tested in humans and may soon become available. Researchers are also working on developing noninvasive blood sugar sensors that would automatically sense blood sugar and, when coupled with an implantable pump would constitute a true, artificial pancreas, delivering appropriate amounts of insulin automatically.

• New surgical techniques have made whole-organ pancreas transplants better than ever. They have been highly successful in restoring blood sugar control to normal, usually in diabetic patients receiving a concurrent kidney transplant to treat kidney failure.

• Transplantation of islet cells, the pancreatic cells that produce insulin, may be available within a few years.

• New drugs have been developed that help treat people with non-insulin-dependent diabetes.

We'll learn more about all of these technologies and discoveries later in this book. Our understanding of diabetes is much more sophisticated and complete than that of the early Greeks, and a great deal of the credit goes to the patients themselves. As can be seen in the Diabetes Control and Complications Trial, patients with diabetes have often volunteered for research studies in the effort to find better ways to treat diabetes.

In a very real sense, everyone who has diabetes becomes something of a scientist. No two people react to the disease, or to treatment, in exactly the same way. Caring for your diabetes will require you to experiment (to a certain extent), to learn about your body, and to learn about yourself. What foods make your blood sugar go up and by how much? How does exercise affect your needs for food and insulin? What happens to your blood sugar levels when you sleep? These are all questions that you will learn how to ask—and how to answer. In the process, you will learn a great deal about how your body works and why.

Diabetes also helps people learn more about themselves as people. The day you found out you had diabetes may have been the most unforgettable of your life, a day when everything changed. Parents whose children are diagnosed often feel the same sort of change; they can't look at anything in the same way anymore. How you deal with your feelings and learn to cope with the disease is just as important as achieving good blood sugar levels. The point of living life, after all, is to enjoy it and be fulfilled. This is just as much a challenge for diabetics as for anyone else with a chronic disease. Each day, that challenge becomes more surmountable, and the disease becomes more a part of a normal, healthy life.

There are two major forms of diabetes. These two forms, one of which is known as type I, or insulin-dependent diabetes mellitus, and the other as type II, or non-insulin-dependent diabetes mellitus, are so different that many doctors almost think of them as "two totally distinct diseases," as Dr. Lynn Levitsky, a pediatric endocrinologist at Mass General, puts it.

That these two distinct entities are commonly called by the same name causes a great deal of confusion. And patients wonder, "Do I need to lose weight?" "Will I need to take insulin?" "Will I be a diabetic all my life?" "Will I ever be able to eat what I want again?" We'll try to answer some of those questions right here.

Insulin-Dependent Diabetes Mellitus (Type I)

When people are learning about diabetes, the first thing that usually confuses them is the terminology. The two principal forms of diabetes used to be called juvenile and adult onset. Juvenile diabetes was usually diagnosed in the young, and adult onset was the type more commonly diagnosed in patients over forty. Then it was discovered that people over forty could have diabetes that was similar to the juvenile form, and young people could develop the adult form. So the two major types of diabetes were renamed type I, or insulin-dependent diabetes mellitus (IDDM), and type II, or non-insulin-dependent diabetes mellitus (NIDDM). Oh, and by the way, just because you're taking insulin doesn't mean that you automatically fall into the first category: you can still have NIDDM, even though you're taking insulin.

Let's try to clear up this confusion. Insulin-dependent diabetes mellitus is caused by an inability to make insulin. Insulin is produced by highly specialized cells in the pancreas called beta cells. IDDM occurs when these beta cells are attacked and destroyed by an autoimmune reaction, a condition in which the body's immune system starts to attack other body cells as if they were foreign invaders. The destruction of your beta cells means that you have no source of insulin. Consequently, you are totally "dependent" on external (or *exogenous,* as you'll often hear) sources of insulin, meaning that in order to stay alive, you require injections of insulin (hence insulin-*dependent* diabetes mellitus). We now know that diabetes is one of a family of related autoimmune diseases, such as Grave's disease (hyperthyroidism), hypothyroidism, Sjögren's disease, rheumatoid arthritis, lupus, and perhaps others. Each of these diseases involves an attack by the immune system on a specific set of human cells. In diabetes, the insulin-producing beta cells in the pancreas are the target of immune destruction. It is not surprising that people with IDDM may also develop other autoimmune diseases, such as hyperthyroidism and hypothyroidism, more commonly than people without diabetes.

The process of destroying the beta cells can take years. In fact, the overt symptoms of diabetes—thirst and frequent urination—usually appear only when you have practically no beta cells left.

As you may have guessed, the lack of insulin presents a severe health problem because insulin is crucial to your body's normal functioning. Your body is composed of many different kinds of cells that have different nutritional requirements for proper operation. Many tissues—particularly skeletal muscle and fat cells—require insulin to transport and utilize glucose (the blood sugar measured by diabetics), their major source of nutrition. In addition, the liver, which acts as a regulator of your nutritional state, is controlled by insulin. When insulin is present or high (for example, after a meal), the liver *stores* dietary sugar and other nutrients; when insulin is low—which occurs in people who are fasting *or* in people with diabetes—the liver synthesizes and releases sugar into the

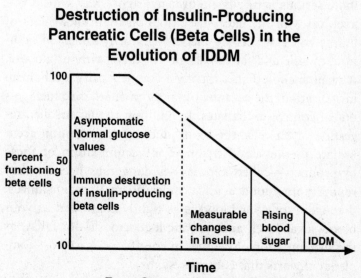

Destruction of Insulin-Producing Pancreatic Cells (Beta Cells) in the Evolution of IDDM

100

Asymptomatic Normal glucose values

Percent functioning beta cells 50

Immune destruction of insulin-producing beta cells

Measurable changes in insulin

Rising blood sugar

IDDM

10

Time From Onset to 10 Years or More

circulation. So, in the absence of insulin, muscle and fat cells can't absorb sugar and the liver pours sugar into the bloodstream. The result is that sugar starts accumulating in the bloodstream, building to levels three, four, even five to ten times as great as normal. At some point, the sugar begins "spilling" into the urine, which is what makes the urine of diabetics sweet. The higher your blood sugar concentration gets, the more you spill into your urine. As the sugar flows into the urine, it takes water with it, which increases urine volume. The resulting frequent urination can lead to dehydration and to increased thirst, which is a kind of protective mechanism. This sequence explains why common first signs of IDDM are frequent urination (*polyuria*) and intense thirst (*polydipsia*).

If the only problems associated with diabetes were thirst and urination, you might not spend a lot of time thinking about it. Unfortunately, problems of a much more serious nature begin brewing right away. Unless you keep up with the excessive urination by drinking lots of fluids, you can become increasingly dehydrated. In addition, muscle and fat cells begin to starve without glucose. A phenomenon that is usually a compensatory mechanism in starvation, the burning of fat as an alternative fuel, gets out of control in diabetes. In addition to uncontrolled digestion of fat cells, the by-products of fat digestion accumulate in the bloodstream. The accumulation of these by-products—called *ketones*—is dangerous because they render your blood acidic. Under normal circumstances, the acidity of your blood is as tightly controlled as your blood sugar level, and diabetic ketoacidosis—or DKA, as the accumulation of ketones in your blood is called—completely thwarts that control system.

DKA is an extremely dangerous condition. In the old

days, before the introduction of insulin, doctors could tell when their diabetic patients were approaching death because their breath would become fruity with the smell of ketones. There was no hope for these children in those pre-insulin days; once in DKA, there was no effective way to prevent them from slipping into a coma and dying soon afterwards.

The discovery of insulin changed all that. Now, if DKA is recognized early, it can be effectively treated with intravenous fluids and insulin. Even more important, most cases of DKA can be prevented by careful monitoring of blood glucose and urine ketone levels, following "sick day" rules, and appropriately adjusting insulin.

Insulin is just one tool the diabetic has to control blood sugar levels, along with diet and exercise. As insulin began to be used in humans, it became clear that a much more comprehensive approach was necessary to keep people with diabetes healthy. Your nondiabetic friends are accustomed to having a pancreas that keeps blood sugar within very tight limits. Their blood sugar levels remain extremely steady, whether they have colds or flus, run marathons, sit all day in front of the television, or even go several days without eating. In any situation, the normal pancreas regulates its secretion of insulin according to the current conditions. It's like breathing; it happens automatically without our thinking about it.

On the other hand, if you have IDDM, you have to think about all these things and plan for all your activities. No matter how tightly you try to control your blood sugar using currently available methods, however, it will never match the exquisite blood sugar regulation provided by a normally functioning pancreas. The lack of truly normal blood sugar control results in both higher and lower than normal levels. Average blood sugar is usually higher than in the non-diabetic person and can result in the long-term complications that we discussed. Later in this book, you'll learn more about how to deal with these complications when they arise. You'll also learn about how to help yourself avoid complications with careful control of blood sugar levels through diet, exercise, and insulin.

Now let's learn a little bit about the other major form of diabetes, non-insulin-dependent diabetes mellitus.

Non-Insulin-Dependent Diabetes Mellitus (Type II)

The major characteristics of non-insulin-dependent diabetes mellitus (NIDDM or type II) are the same as insulin-dependent diabetes mellitus (IDDM): elevated blood sugar levels and long-term complications. However, the cause of these elevated blood sugar levels, the acute metabolic complications, and therapies are quite different.

IDDM starts with destruction of the beta cells in the pancreas. No beta cells, no insulin. No insulin, no normal human metabolism. On the other hand, patients with NIDDM often produce lots and lots of insulin. The problem they have is twofold. One problem usually lies in their responsiveness or, more accurately, their decreased responsiveness to the insulin they produce. NIDDM patients are usually "insulin resistant." This means that insulin is less effective at lowering blood sugar levels. The causes of insulin resistance in NIDDM are multiple, but a common factor is that most people with NIDDM—usually more than 80 percent—are overweight. Bigger people need more insulin.

The second problem leading to NIDDM is *relatively*

low (compared with similar weight non-diabetes) insulin secretion, and this explains why only about 20 to 25 percent of overweight people ever develop diabetes. Those overweight people who develop NIDDM are people who can't make enough insulin to meet their elevated demand.

Although blood sugar levels may often be as high in persons with NIDDM as in IDDM, they tend to rise more slowly over time after diabetes develops. This may explain why patients with NIDDM tend to have fewer symptoms of hyperglycemia, as high blood sugar is known, compared with patients with IDDM. In fact, many patients with NIDDM have few if any symptoms, which leads to almost one half of the NIDDM population not even knowing they have diabetes. The absence of symptoms, however, doesn't mean that NIDDM patients are out of danger. Far from it: NIDDM is associated with all of the long-term eye, kidney, and nerve problems as occur in IDDM. In addition, people with NIDDM are usually obese and have high blood pressure and abnormal levels of blood cholesterol and other circulating blood lipids. The abnormal blood cholesterol, blood pressure, and blood sugar levels place these people at markedly elevated risk for heart disease.

There are several ways for many people with NIDDM to *control their blood sugar levels without using insulin*. The first is weight control, whether through diet, exercise, or both. While this sounds relatively easy, it turns out to be very difficult for many people with NIDDM to control their weight. In this book, we'll hear from people who are trying or have tried to control their diabetes by reducing their weight.

The second method for people with NIDDM to control their blood sugar without insulin injections is through the use of oral agents that can raise the level of insulin production by the pancreas, decrease sugar production by the liver, or decrease the rate of sugar absorption from the intestine. We'll learn more about how these oral agents work and their advantages and disadvantages later in this book (see Chapter 10).

If you have NIDDM, what's most important is that you realize the seriousness of your condition and treat it accordingly. Many people with NIDDM profess to feeling just fine, despite their high blood sugars, and they refuse to recognize the long-term dangers of neglecting to seek proper medical attention. Anyone who does this is taking a big risk: NIDDM predisposes you to much higher rates of cardiovascular disease than are found in the non-diabetic population, as well as the serious diabetic complications of kidney disease, eye disease, and nervous system dysfunction. The same lessons learned in the DCCT for persons with IDDM almost certainly apply in NIDDM— glucose control matters and people with diabetes who maintain lower blood sugar levels will be more likely to escape the long-term complications.

Other Forms of Diabetes

A third, less well known type of diabetes is called GDM, or gestational diabetes mellitus. Men don't need to worry about GDM, at least not on their own behalf, because it occurs only in pregnant women.

GDM usually begins during the last trimester in approximately 5 percent of all pregnancies and usually disappears after delivery. However, 30 to 50 percent of women with GDM go on to develop NIDDM later in life. Another important reason for you to be aware of GDM is that it is associated with higher rates of complications during delivery and in the newborn. As we'll see in Chapter 9, it's important for women with GDM to seek out experienced help promptly and restore their blood sugar levels to a normal range. All pregnant women are supposed to be screened for GDM between the twenty-fourth and twenty-eighth week of pregnancy. If you have had GDM with a previous pregnancy, you might be screened even earlier in your pregnancy.

There are other, less common causes of diabetes that we seldom hear about. These include:

- Diabetes as a result of pancreatic diseases such as pancreatitis, pancreatic cancer, cystic fibrosis, and hemochromatosis.
- Diabetes induced by chemicals or drugs such as glucocorticoids (steroids) or thiazide diuretics (commonly used to treat hypertension).
- Diabetes associated with genetic syndromes such as Turner's syndrome, myotonic dystrophy, and Prader-Willi syndrome.
- Diabetes resulting from rare abnormalities in insulin, the cellular receptor for the insulin molecule, and an autosomal dominant, inherited form of diabetes (passed from generation to generation to about half the children of affected parents) that is caused by an abnormal pancreatic protein that results in decreased insulin release.

The common theme running through all these forms of diabetes—IDDM, NIDDM, and all these others—is that, despite all our knowledge and all the best research in the best hospitals of the world, diabetes remains an extremely difficult disease to cope with. People with diabetes continue to feel alienated and alone. Many of them are afraid or reluctant to seek out the knowledge and medical attention that can help them control their diabetes, either because they're afraid that they may have to abandon old habits of eating or activity, or because they don't want to be treated differently.

This book is designed to help you find your way through these obstacles to better health. You'll hear from health care professionals—doctors, nurses, dietitians, and others—about how they view diabetes, how they treat it, and what they consider the best approaches to health in diabetes. And you'll also hear from all kinds of people with diabetes. We'll speak with those who have had diabetes for years without complications. We'll also hear from those who have suffered through complications such as blindness, heart disease, and kidney disease. You'll hear the stories of transplant patients. And you'll also listen to the words of diabetic children and their parents.

Dealing with diabetes may never be easy, any more than dealing with any chronic illness, but hearing from other patients who have walked down the same road can be helpful. I hope that you'll take comfort and inspiration from the stories of others who will share their successes, and their failures, of coping with diabetes.

2

Diagnosis

Some morning, you've probably awoken to feel a little scratch in your throat. You were snuffling a little bit each time you breathed, and you guessed it was only allergies or just some dust in the air. Maybe, you hoped, it would just go away.

A few hours later, you knew that it wasn't allergies. Your head was pounding and you felt achy all over. At that point you knew that you were in for a few unpleasant days.

"Damn," you thought with resignation. "I've got a cold." It meant limiting your activity for a couple of days, drinking lots of liquids, and "taking care of yourself" with lots of sleep, acetaminophen or aspirin, and perhaps chicken soup. Looking out at what the next week or so held was not the most enjoyable prospect, because you had to limit your activity, but at least there was an end in sight.

That you were suffering from a cold was obvious to you and everyone around you, and everyone was prepared with instructions about how to treat it. Friends would tell you about their favorite home remedies—keep your head warm, eat lots of garlic, take vitamin C—all the while looking over your shoulder to make sure that you followed their advice. Because if you didn't, and your cold got worse, they would have reason to say, "Look at that. Didn't take care of himself, and now he's worse than ever." In other words, "I told you so."

When you "awaken" to find you have diabetes, a similar process takes place, but in this case it's much more acute. First of all, you probably didn't know what was happening when you first experienced the symptoms of diabetes. You knew that something was amiss, that much was clear. Getting up three, four, or five times a night to go to the bathroom; being tired and sleepy all day long; drinking everything in sight. One of my patients, a nurse, recalled a trip that she took days before her diagnosis with NIDDM. She was on her way to a friend's wedding in Pennsylvania, and she had to stop the car every fifteen minutes to go to the bathroom. On her way back to the car, she would stop at the "filling station" to buy a soda—and drink the whole thing before she even opened the car door! She knew something was wrong, but even with her background in nursing, she was unable to identify it.

Some people are not unhappy with the very early signs of diabetes; these are usually people who are pleased to be losing lots of weight, since, without adequate insulin levels, they are unable to absorb the glucose and other nutrients (see Chapter 1). But as these other symptoms, such as frequent urination (doctors call it *polyuria*) and unquenchable thirst *(polydipsia)* worsen, most people will eventually recognize that it's time to see a doctor.

After hearing a patient history that includes weight loss, polyuria, and polydipsia, almost any doctor will immediately suspect diabetes. The test for diabetes is simple. In fact, at least one mother I know diagnosed her own daughter's diabetes at home. Carmella Clark has had IDDM herself since the age of ten. Her one-year-old daughter, Jessie, was "drinking around six bottles at night. She was constantly waking up and urinating, and was constantly getting rashes."

After several days of trying to understand what was wrong, Carmella decided to use her own monitor to test Jessie's blood sugar. The result: 513 mg/dl, well out of the range of normal human blood sugar levels (normally between about 70 and 115 mg/dl after fasting and less than 180 after eating), and indicative of diabetes. And, basically, that was it. There might be a number of medical reasons for a one-year-old to have recurrent rashes, and several reasons for her to be thirsty and frequently urinating. But the combination of all these symptoms and the elevated blood sugar made the diagnosis of diabetes a cinch.

I'm not suggesting that diabetes is best diagnosed in the home. On the contrary, doctors have the best equipment and knowledge to make the diagnosis and to advise a person who has suddenly found that diabetes is about to become a lifelong companion. Carmella happened to have the equipment on hand and decided to use it. But if you suspect, or even discover, as Carmella did, that you or someone you know has diabetes, get to a doctor as soon as possible.

Although endocrinologists (internists who specialize in hormonal diseases) and diabetologists (endocrinologists who focus on diabetes) may be best equipped to treat IDDM, all internists, family practitioners, and general practitioners should be able to diagnose diabetes and initiate therapy. NIDDM is so common that all physicians help to take care of it.

The diagnosis of diabetes is really quite simple. There is a classic "constellation" of signs and symptoms that doctors look for, including the features we've already talked about—polyuria, polydipsia, weight loss—and some others, including frequent eating *(polyphagia)*. In the presence of these symptoms, any blood sugar over 200 mg/dl is indicative of diabetes.

People with NIDDM may exhibit some of these symptoms, but not at a level that makes them suspect anything is wrong. That is, they might get up in the middle of the night to urinate, and they might sense they're a little more thirsty than usual, but nothing beyond that. However, if you're overweight and more than forty-five years old, ask yourself a couple of questions: How much exercise do I get? Do any of my blood relatives have diabetes? If you get little or no exercise, and people in your family have diabetes, then you may be at risk. In that case, it is worth talking to your physician about being screened for diabetes. In addition, if you are an African American, Hispanic American, American Indian, or an Asian or Pacific Island American, you are at even higher risk than Caucasian Americans. Finally, any woman with a past history of GDM should be followed carefully.

Diabetes is diagnosed if two blood sugar measurements are greater than 140 mg/dl in a patient who has fasted overnight. Alternatively, a second test, called the *oral glucose tolerance test,* allows the doctor to detemine whether diabetes is present. In this test, which is used infrequently,

75 grams of glucose—in the form of a sugary cola syrup—is given to a fasting patient. If the two-hour blood sugar is greater than 200 mg/dl, diabetes is probably present. In fact, most NIDDM develops with rising post-prandial (after eating) blood sugar levels, followed by rising fasting sugar levels.

The time immediately after diagnosis is very difficult and very important for people with diabetes. Many people find it emotionally draining to confront their disease. "Why me?" is a question we often hear from patients and one for which we have few satisfactory answers.

"You look in the mirror and nothing has changed," said one patient. "How can it be that I suddenly have diabetes?"

Rather than accept their condition, some people deny that they have diabetes and refuse to deal with it. To confuse matters more, many people with IDDM experience something called a *honeymoon phase* immediately after diagnosis. During the honeymoon phase, the symptoms of diabetes and the need for insulin may all but disappear. Why the honeymoon phase occurs is still a matter of much debate, but the effect that it has on patients can be quite wrenching. Patients often believe that their diagnosis was some kind of mistake and that they don't have diabetes after all. Their relief may translate into reckless behavior that may result in high blood sugars, which can have disastrous short- and long-term consequences. Most doctors prepare their newly diagnosed patients with IDDM for the honeymoon phase, but some patients are fooled by it and have to adjust themselves to the reality of diabetes all over again.

Christian DiRomualdo was diagnosed with diabetes at the age of one year. When I spoke with his parents, Nancy and Tony, Christian appeared to be coming out of his honeymoon phase, and his sugars were shooting up over 300 mg/dl.

"His sugars have been really erratic over the past couple of weeks," said Tony. "It's made us realize that he is not going to spend the rest of his life at the current insulin dosage. It's going to increase as he gets bigger."

The experience of being diagnosed with diabetes is different for almost everyone. To some, it is a crushing blow, an obstacle that is never completely overcome. Some people never really accept their diabetes and never really treat it properly or responsibly. Some lean on family and friends to take care of their diabetes for them: a short-term solution that can carry them briefly, but not for a whole life. But a great many people learn to accept their diabetes, to understand it, to cope with it and to incorporate it into their lives, without fear. These people—and there are many of them—find that diabetes is something they can live with. It is not the end of the world, the end of life as they know it, the final curtain on all that is enjoyable in life.

Wendy Avery Smith had been diagnosed with diabetes twenty-six years ago, when she was eleven years old. Although she took care of her diabetes, she never really became obsessed with self-care until she found that she was pregnant. Her attitude has always been one of quiet coping.

"My concept of this is not that I'm an ill person," Wendy told me. "There's a hormone that my body doesn't provide, insulin, and I have to do extra things to make up for it. The stereotypical definition of chronic illness doesn't fit me; there are not many things I can't do, except maybe fly an airplane."

After having known countless patients with diabetes, I would say that the most common characteristic of people who do well with diabetes is their willingness to learn and adjust. They see their lives and habits as changeable. They look at situations with flexibility and optimism, and they view obstacles as surmountable. They have a strong desire for a healthy life and freedom from complications, and they are willing to work hard and sacrifice to attain those things.

Kathy Hurxthal, a nurse educator with many years of experience in Mass General's Diabetes Clinic, is often the first person to see people after they've been diagnosed with diabetes. Here is Kathy's approach to dealing with people right after they've been diagnosed:

- "We make an effort to be as simple as possible the first time we talk to newly diagnosed patients. Roughly, what we recommend is that they have three meals a day, eat less fat, eat less refined or pure sugar, and keep a diet diary.

- "We ask them for a 24-hour dietary recall and calculate what they're taking in and expending in terms of calories. Then we can use that to make diet recommendations and set insulin dosage. We'll try to encourage patients not to worry about their diet at first. Improving the diet, if it's necessary, is something that has to be done gradually and naturally.

- "We talk to patients about medications, and we try to stress that even if they're taking pills rather than insulin, they still may be at risk for episodes of low blood sugar. These can be dangerous, so we make sure that they have some blood sugar testing skills. We find that that's something patients want to learn how to do, they want to find out what their blood sugar levels are, and that's the first step in getting control of them.

• "Often, people are in a state of shock immediately after being diagnosed with diabetes. I remember an eighteen-year-old girl who was a student here in Boston. She went home for a brief vacation, and while she was home, she had a blood sugar of 600 and was feeling dry and thirsty. She had to come back to school, and her mother, who was frantic, decided to send her to Mass General. The daughter was forced to learn very quickly about how to take care of her diabetes, while at the same time she was adjusting to life at school. It took a while for it to sink in that we were talking about a change in her body that would affect the rest of her life.

• "I've often found myself telling newly diagnosed people, 'You're going to hear a lot of things from a lot of people. People will come out of the woodwork giving advice.' Diabetes is all over the place—one out of every ten people have diabetes at some time in their lives. So everyone knows someone who has diabetes, and because of that experience they think they know everything about the disease. You have to stick to your guns, stick to your own treatment team's recommendations and your own treatment plan. Don't be swayed by people who want to tell you all about an uncle with diabetes who ate one donut in 1956 and died.

• "With the publication of results from the Diabetes Control and Complications Trial (DCCT), we have something really very important to tell them. Several years ago, there was some question as to whether good blood sugar control made any difference in the development of complications. Well, those questions have been answered, and the controversy has been laid to rest. Now we can tell people with diabetes to try as hard as they can to keep their blood sugars under control. Chances are very good that this will save them from having to deal with some hard-to-handle complications like blindness and kidney failure, and it may help them live longer. Now we've got more ammunition to help convince people to try as hard as they can." (You'll learn more about the DCCT later in Chapters 4 to 6, and 10.)

It's not unusual for family members to react strongly to the diagnosis of diabetes, sometimes more dramatically or irrationally than the patients themselves. At times, a family member will openly deny the fact of diabetes, just as people who have been diagnosed do, and insist that nothing has changed. Parents, in particular, have a tendency to mourn when their children are diagnosed with diabetes. Not long ago, I spoke with a diabetes specialist whose child had been diagnosed with the disease several years ago. I asked her whether, with her knowledge and qualifications for teaching her son about diabetes, it was any easier to accept this turn of events. As I posed the question, her eyes lowered and her face hardened.

"Not at all," she replied, without taking time to think. "I was devastated when I found out that Bill was going to have to deal with this. I know all too well what diabetes means, what it can do."

Gail Denman was diagnosed when she was nine. Her mother had been diabetic since her own childhood and had managed her own diabetes extremely well. Therefore, Gail had never had a life completely without diabetes. However, she had never felt herself crushed by her diagnosis. Her mother, on the other hand, felt extremely guilty for having "passed the disease along" to her daughter.

Childbearing is one of the most emotionally volatile experiences of our lives, and, as parents, each of us takes responsibility for the shape and quality of our children's bodies and for their health. How often we say something like, "She has your eyes, but my mouth." The parents of diabetic children have a tendency to look at their offspring and say, "She has my pancreas; my inherited defect." In reality, diabetes inheritance patterns are very poorly understood, and any geneticist will tell you that there is no scientific sense and certainly nothing to be gained by blaming yourself for your child's diabetes.

Gail's mother began to feel even worse when Gail's eyesight began failing in her mid-twenties. This was a development no one had expected, and it has changed the relationship between Gail and her mother in a significant and seemingly permanent way. At her home, Gail proudly showed me pictures of her mother, a beautiful woman who has lived with diabetes since well before the time of precise blood glucose testing methods. Gail's mother was and is a great walker; she walks everywhere she can, and uses this exercise, along with insulin and diet, to help keep her blood sugars in a near-normal range. This has probably contributed greatly to her good health over the years. But she has had great difficulty confronting Gail's complications, which she sees as a failing on her part, a biological failure, and perhaps a failure as a mother.

Somewhat surprisingly, there are people who feel as though their diagnosis of diabetes has benefited their lives in some way. One of my patients once told me that diabetes came at a time in her life when she needed to become more organized and self-controlled. Diabetes demanded that she do that, and she complied.

"Much of the time I feel as if I am really lucky that I have diabetes," says Ralph Dineen, a Boston architect with IDDM. "I know that sounds weird. But what I mean by that is because of my diabetes, and through my diabetes, I have paid more attention to my general health than I would have otherwise. I suppose it sounds fatalistic, but suppose I had continued with my old eating habits: I could have developed colon cancer or heart disease, because I wouldn't have paid attention to my diet.

"I consider that I am very lucky that I have diabetes because it is something that I can manage. I couldn't say that at the onset of the disease, but I can say it now because when I was diagnosed, I entered a kind of compact with myself about my diabetes. I determined my own willingness to participate in a hands-on way—and I *can* do that. My mother-in-law died of ovarian cancer, and there was not a thing I or anyone else could do to help her, nor that she could do to help herself. I consider myself pretty fortunate to have such a manageable disease, if that is what I am going to be blessed with. So, in a weird sort of way, diabetes is good news."

As I've said, diabetes is a great teacher, and Ralph's words point out one of the continuing lessons I've learned through treating people with diabetes. There are many tools for treating the disease, but certainly one of the most effective is a positive attitude, especially when this includes a willingness to take the best out of life. Ralph acknowledges that at the time he was diagnosed, life didn't look as rosy as it may have in the past. But he survived that difficult time and found that much more rewarding things lay for him around the corner, that his disease could even afford him a sense of security.

This level of acceptance of diabetes is something that

takes a person quite some time to achieve. Many people may need counseling at the time of diagnosis. Patients are vulnerable to fears about the future, to feelings of isolation and being incomplete, to feelings of inadequacy. Carol Wool, a psychiatrist at Mass General who specializes in working with people with chronic conditions, says that people with diabetes often feel less than whole, and they find shame and humiliation in being different.

"They say, 'I can't tell anyone. I don't want anyone to know that I have to eat at noon,' " Carol says. "At first they don't want anyone to kid them, they only want to fit in. But there's always a sense that they don't fit in, and because of that differentness there's a rift. Over the long term, some people will surmount that rift and start to see themselves as legitimate members of the community again. But others feel very alone."

The time of diagnosis is no time to feel alone, and if you have recently been diagnosed, make sure that you reach out to your friends and family. Tell them how you want to be treated, whether you consider it an open topic for discussion or whether it makes you more comfortable to treat it quietly. It's useful to contact the American Diabetes Association (ADA); your local chapter may be able to give you the names of other association members who will talk to you about diabetes and calm your fears about what the future holds for you.

The same sense of dread that makes diabetes so difficult to deal with—fear of the unknown—makes many people hesitant to consult a psychiatrist or similar professional at times like these. If you feel fear or distaste about this kind of care, try to overcome it; talking about your feelings about the diagnosis can help you confront and cope with them. Make use of the resources around you, and start dealing with your diabetes as soon as possible. When you do, you'll find that living with diabetes is something that you can do—even if it doesn't happen overnight—and that will give you a tremendous sense of self-satisfaction.

3

The Treatment Team

When talking about the diabetes treatment team, it's very easy to roll out all the clichés about "team spirit," and "giving it all you've got," and "everyone depends on everyone else." And there are some similarities between the team that helps you take care of your diabetes and, say, a baseball team: both are collections of people with specialized skills, and each team works together toward its common goal.

But in one important aspect, your diabetes treatment team is very different. They say that a lawyer will walk in and out of the courtroom by your side—but won't go to jail with you. Well, it's the same with your treatment team. Most of the time—but certainly not all of the time—you're the only one on your treatment team who actually *has* diabetes. You are the only one who can put your treatment plan into play. And if your treatment plan fails, your treatment team will, of course, sympathize with you and offer support, but you will be the only one harmed.

As we've seen from the results of the Diabetes Control and Complications Trial, it's of crucial importance for people with diabetes to keep tight control over their blood sugar to avoid complications. Tightly controlled blood sugar levels can help you stave off the neuropathy, kidney disease, and eye disease that attend diabetes, perhaps avoiding them indefinitely.

One of our central assumptions in setting up the DCCT was that in order to get safe and effective intensive treatment, people with diabetes should be under the care of a treatment team, one that ideally includes a diabetologist (an M.D. who specializes in diabetes), a diabetes nurse educator, and a dietitian. You need a treatment team that can help you keep your blood sugar under control and do it without driving you crazy. It's common for people with diabetes to feel guilty about and alone with their disease. They can find it hard to reach out to others and talk about their problems. Some find it difficult to be honest about their self-treatment. Others feel overwhelmed by the seemingly enormous responsibilities of taking care of their own health, and they abdicate the burden of their diabetes.

In short, there are all kinds of responses to diabetes, and a good treatment team should help you deal with them. Let's meet some of the people on Mass General's treatment team, see what they think of the work they do, why they do it, and what they can do for you.

The Diabetologist

I came to diabetes treatment and clinical research via the laboratory. After training in internal medicine, I specialized in endocrinology, the study of the human body's glands and the hormones, like insulin, that they secrete. More interested in how things work than how to fix them, I looked forward happily to a life in research. Quite suddenly, the chief of the diabetes unit departed, and I was asked to take the job of directing diabetes clinical research and care. It was an interesting time in diabetes, a time of great potential, when the ability to treat and control diabetes, to prevent complications, and to reverse their progression, was really growing. I accepted and became director of the Diabetes Clinical Research Center and Clinic at Massachusetts General Hospital.

I would like to say that I have always had insight into clinical diabetes, but I'm not sure that I did early on. However, endocrinology has always been a science-driven subspecialty and new research tools have always benefited our clinical understanding. In fact, the first substance measured by radioimmunoassay was insulin, and the first gene to be cloned was the gene for insulin.

The scientific aspects of endocrinology drew me to the field, and to diabetes in particular. When you're studying a specific disease, it's convenient to have a lot of patients, and diabetes is obviously a very common disease. Of course, you can study rare diseases in great detail and learn important lessons from them, but the practical applications of those studies may be limited. And I have always been especially interested in the practical applications of my research; I study diabetes not only to solve its puzzles and satisfy my curiosity, but in hope of helping people who suffer from the disease.

I see myself as performing a variety of functions for the patient. First of all, I'm the patient's link with the health care system, often serving as a primary care physician. There are few, if any, medical issues for my diabetes patients in which I do not get involved or have some say. I also am a referral center, deciding when the patient should see, for instance, Dr. Nina Rubin, the nephrologist (kidney specialist), Kathy Hurxthal, the diabetes nurse educator, or Linda Delahanty, one of the dietitians who specializes in diabetes.

The care of people with diabetes is really a team, or ensemble, effort, with the patient playing the leading role and the professional staff playing supporting roles. For patients with IDDM (insulin-dependent diabetes mellitus), intensive therapy has become the accepted mode of therapy for the present and the future, and it may be shown to be the therapy of choice for patients with NIDDM (non-insulin-dependent diabetes mellitus), too. To make it work, intensively treated patients need an incredible amount of input from dietitians and diabetes educators. The whole team has to stay involved.

I'm used to seeing people have trouble coping emotionally with their diabetes. And while I use my knowledge of diabetes and its treatment to help patients understand and treat fluctuations in blood sugar levels with adjustments in their insulin, diet, and exercise regimen, I also try to impart the bigger picture, describing their condition in the context of the rest of their lives.

As I see each person, I try to keep a number of factors in mind when determining how to help them deal with their diabetes. What is his or her level of understanding? Can this person comply with a rigorous treatment plan? What is his or her general health like? Will treating one problem potentially exacerbate others? For example, if the person has cardiovascular disease, will treating the heart problem affect diabetes? There are probably hundreds of things that a doctor has to keep in mind when seeing and thinking about each patient, and although it would be useful, it's probably impossible to reduce it all to one easy set of rules for treatment. If doctors find themselves challenged by the complexity of diabetes, think how difficult it must be for the patient.

There is a set of consensus recommendations for treatment available from the ADA (American Diabetes Association). As someone who contributed to its development, I think it's not bad. But do I think it is always the most efficient and cost-effective way of treating people with diabetes? Well, no. The recommendations may be generally correct, but they may not apply to a particular patient. And like many diabetologists, I have my own personal "flow chart" based on our own studies here at Mass General and individualized for each patient. According to *that* flow chart, I ask myself, does this patient need to see an ophthalmologist this year? A podiatrist (foot specialist), or a cardiologist? How will he or she react to this medicine, or a change in insulin schedule?

You can't send patients off to specialists in an automatic, predetermined fashion, just because a consensus recommendation says you should. And there are many times when a patient needs special attention, and there's no flow chart in the world that can tell you when and why. I suppose all of our decisions could be computerized, removing the fallibility of human decision making. But I wonder if it would be better? The bottom line is that the care we provide and organize for the patient, and the lessons we teach, are only a small part of diabetes care. The majority of diabetes treatment, hour-to-hour and day-to-day, is self-care. And as complex as we think our part of the management is, the patient's role is infinitely more complicated.

Dr. John Godine, one of my colleagues here at Mass General's Diabetes Unit, uses a computer to follow (not to treat) his patients. The computer is actually no more than a little day-minder—he calls it a "pocket brain"—that he uses to record the daily blood sugar readings of some peo-ple whose diabetes is more "brittle," or prone to fluctua-tion. Dr. Godine enjoys treating people with diabetes because of its never-ending complexity and the similarities it holds to primary care, and because of the ties that en-docrinology holds to other disciplines in medicine, like cardiology, neurology, and nephrology.

The pocket brain allows Dr. Godine to carry around in-formation that he can't necessarily hold inside his head. It's an organizational tool, but it can't make decisions for him about how to treat a patient's diabetes. Similarly, he tries to give people information that will be helpful to them in treating their own diabetes, but he can't actually organize them or their lives.

In response to the seemingly impossible task of orga-nizing their lives, some patients respond to diabetes by making themselves into "food robots." Wary of experi-menting with foods, and terrified of running very high or low blood sugars, they eat exactly the same diet every day, so that their insulin needs remain constant. It takes some of the guesswork and uncertainty out of diabetes, but it takes a lot of the fun out of life, too.

On the other hand, Godine concedes that there are many people who aren't comfortable with being organized or can't manage it, and there may be no way to get them to enjoy having order in their lives. "I try to help people organize themselves, but I'm not sure I succeed," he says. For some people, the response that is most comfortable turns out to be the most productive, and for others it isn't.

In at least one respect, it may be fortunate that so many people with IDDM are diagnosed at a young age, because it gives their parents, doctors, and other health care per-sonnel the opportunity to help them cultivate organiza-tional skills, take pride in the self-care of their diabetes, and avoid acquiring the type of random eating, sleeping, and exercise habits that make it difficult to care for diabetes later in life. Dr. Lynne Levitsky, director of pediatric endocrinology at Mass General, points out that patients with newly diagnosed diabetes are like clean slates, ready to learn techniques and principles of self-management; patients who have already learned "bad habits," on the other hand, are frequently even more of a challenge. I asked her for some perspective on the diverse ways that she helps parents whose children have diabetes.

"Well, besides applying clinical knowledge, we try to intervene with good parenting skills," Dr. Levitsky says. "That includes listening, praising things that are good, trying to keep as open as possible with the family. Pediatricians do a lot of things that are like good parenting.

"In some cases, we have developed courses intended to help parents deal with issues related to diabetes. We try to help them enforce consistency, and when we see problems, we try to counsel people as best we can. Many destructive behaviors are hard to eradicate. For instance, there are many parents who worry that every time they say no, they are warping their children for life. So they intermittently say yes and no, and the best way to reinforce an unwanted behavior in a child is to give contradictory messages."

Doctors who treat diabetes often find themselves in a frustrating position. They want to help you, the patient, stay healthy, and very often they can tell you how to get to that state of health. And patients are often very receptive to the counsel they get from their doctors. Enthusiasm, however, for aggressive self-treatment can wane quickly as patients confront the demands of self-care. The challenge to diabetologists is to discover what motivates their patients, to see the best in them, and turn that power toward achieving the highest level of health possible.

"You're in the role of giving a lot of advice," says Levitsky. "People who go into endocrinology usually do so because they like diagnosing weird diseases, not because they enjoy chronic lifestyle–preventive medicine interaction, which is what primary care providers should be doing but can't because they see forty patients a day. And in diabetes, that's what you're doing—a tremendous amount of it. It's like primary care, but there's no financial reimbursement for the time you spend. The pleasure of treating diabetes is watching children develop and grow, and watching families mature, and seeing things go right.

"The therapeutic challenges are unmet and endless. I happen to like that, and if I didn't, I would probably leave the field. And that would probably be pretty painful because I'm so intensely involved in my work. I've talked to dietitians and they feel the same way: you walk out of a morning clinic when you've seen six or seven kids with diabetes, and you feel drained, as though you've had a long workout. And then you look at the families of the patients, and they feel that way *all the time.* They are asking questions we have no answers to. They desperately want their kids to live long, happy lives and not to develop long-term complications. They know what it takes to get there, and they know that they can get there with the tools they have today. But they're frustrated because they want us to look at what they're doing and magically come up with answers that they don't have and we don't have."

The Diabetes Nurse Educator

When Kathy Hurxthal was a young girl, she used to go to the hospital to visit her father, who was a busy practicing endocrinologist with a research interest in thyroid disease. There were always things for her to do around the office and the laboratory; sometimes, her father would use her in clinical studies, perhaps to provide a blood sample. Occasionally, she would talk with her father about the most common and costly of endocrinologic diseases, diabetes.

In addition to being an endocrinologist, Dr. Lewis Hurxthal had diabetes himself, non-insulin dependent. He probably diagnosed himself in his mid-fifties, his daughter said. Dr. Hurxthal was not one to let diabetes get in the way of living; in addition to a full clinical practice, teaching, and research, he was an avid gardener and painter, and he pursued these latter activities vigorously until his death at the age of eighty-six, despite mild complications of cataracts and neuropathy. This should come as no surprise; many people with diabetes live into their seventies and eighties, and we'll meet more of them in this book. Like many successfully self-managed people with diabetes, Dr. Hurxthal was not modest about having the disease, and he made no attempt to disguise it in front of either his colleagues or his family. He often administered his pre-meal insulin at the dinner table.

Hurxthal followed in her father's footsteps in a number of ways—in painting and in patient care. But where the father had been a doctor, the daughter pursued a career as a nurse. Kathy became more and more interested in caring for patients with diabetes. After working for several years in ward nursing, she studied to become a diabetes nurse educator. The idea of a treatment team that included a diabetes nurse educator was not widespread when she started doing it. The first meeting of her professional society in 1978 barely filled a small meeting hall. Since then, the American Diabetes Association has recognized and endorsed the crucial nature of education in diabetes care, and the profession has grown to include thousands of specialists.

The diabetes nurse educator is an extremely important member of the treatment team and often the person who solidifies the link between the team and the patient. Sooner or later, many outpatients treated for diabetes at Mass General walk through her door and sit down. She's a teacher, a motivator, a constant source of advice, sometimes a confessor when patients want to talk about their "transgressions," and often the person patients speak with when their doctors are not immediately available. She's frequently the first person on the treatment team to see people with diabetes after they're diagnosed, and she will teach them how to perform self-monitoring and to self-administer their first insulin injection. The first name that diabetic patients often mention at Mass General is Kathy Hurxthal's.

In her first meeting with a patient, Kathy Hurxthal usually tries to get across a few basic points about self-management that every diabetic should know:

• Consistency. Try to eat, exercise, and take insulin on a regular schedule. Three meals and one or two snacks a day are the norm. Inject your insulin, or take your medication, at consistent times.

• Moderation. Limit fat and sugar in the diet. No one can go through life without eating fat or sugar, but for the sake of your health, it's worthwhile to learn how to read a food label and prepare healthy meals.

• Self-awareness. Keep a diary of diet and blood sugar readings. Know how many calories you're taking in, and

plan how you're going to cover them with exercise and insulin (see Chapters 5 and 6).

• Control. You're in charge of your diabetes. People
will come out of the woodwork to give advice. While it
never hurts to listen politely, you need to work with your
treatment team to develop a plan for dealing with your diabetes, and then stick to it.

These are only the most preliminary starting rules for
the person with diabetes. They have many lessons to learn,
including how to monitor and take medication; how to
prevent hypoglycemia (low blood sugar) and treat it
should it occur; how to cope with "sick days"; the fine
points of dietary management; the goals of diabetes care;
foot care; and many others. Luckily not all of them need
to be taught at once.

Kathy believes that motivation is one of the most important issues for people with diabetes. Finding better
ways to get them excited about treating themselves is
something that everyone on the treatment team faces. Diabetes is a lifelong disease, and patients constantly need a
source of energy to keep them excited about maintaining
their good health and treating their disease.

"If you had a secret bullet that would get people moti-
vated, that would be great," Kathy says. "You can try fear,
but it doesn't work, usually. Sometimes we make contracts
with patients, an agreement that says that if you get a certain amount of exercise and maintain a certain blood
sugar level, then you can have these foods. Or you can
work with guilt; you can say, 'Take care of yourself, if not
for yourself, then because your children need you.' There's
no way of telling what the most effective way is."

Kathy deals with all kinds of requests for information:

she teaches patients how and where to give themselves their insulin or diabetes medications; she addresses people's misconceptions about diabetes, such as the common idea that it is caused by eating too many sweets; she watches patients go through the grieving process that often takes place after the diagnosis of diabetes, and she tries to help them cope. When a workplace situation, perhaps a long afternoon meeting that conflicts with a snack, puts a patient in danger of suffering an insulin reaction, Kathy is often the first to hear about it. She spends time with patients describing the short-term and long-term complications of diabetes, and how to avoid them with tight blood sugar control, and she helps patients find doctors to give preventive care and treat complications when they do arise. She likes it when patients come in with a list of questions or concerns, so that she can deal fully with as many sources of anxiety as possible.

Sometimes, patients' problems are of a psychological nature, yet are so particular to diabetes that the involvement of the diabetes educator can help. Leah Berthold, a pediatric diabetes educator, can recall many times when this has been true. In fact, very frequently it is the parents of the newly diagnosed diabetic child who have trouble coming to terms with the disease. For instance, one young girl was in the hospital for two extra days because her mother was having difficulty giving the insulin injections. Two days doesn't seem like a long time, Berthold points out, but most parents learn to give the injections within a day. Berthold suspected that the mother's inability to accept her daughter's illness was the root of the problem.

Dealing with problems like this become part of the nurse educator's job; it's a wide-ranging one that demands lots of contact with patients and their families, and empathy for their problems. No other area of medicine requires such an intimate knowledge of the patient's lifestyle and day-to-day activities.

The Dietitian

We are surrounded by food. Every other television ad, billboard, book, newspaper article, every other word coming out of every other person's mouth has something to do with food.

After language, the most important component of any culture is probably its food. The poet T. S. Eliot refused to journey to China, he said, because he had no interest in a country without a native cheese. "You are what you eat," we are often reminded, perhaps suggesting that a simple reduction in food intake would diminish us as human beings. (I wonder if this underlies the epidemic of obesity?)

So you have diabetes. What does that mean? Is someone going to walk into your kitchen, unplug the refrigerator, take it away and never bring it back? In Shakespeare's *Twelfth Night,* Sir Toby says to the clown, "Dost thou think that because thou art virtuous, there shall be no more cakes and ale?" Well, rest assured that the post-diagnosis era will contain opportunities for cakes and ale. The only difference is that these cakes and ale will be planned for and consumed in the context of a diabetic regimen.

Linda Delahanty, a Mass General dietitian who specializes in diabetes care, tries to assist patients with that kind of planning. Her job is to help people understand the connection between what they're eating and their blood sugar levels and weight. Many patients think that her goal is to get them to surrender their favorite foods, but that's not the case, Delahanty says.

"In the old days," she recalls, talking about a time less than ten or fifteen years ago, "you were given a certain insulin or medication prescription, and it was expected that your diet would be worked around it. We were trying to mold habits around that prescription, and if you know anything about habits, you know how difficult they are to change. Now we're going the opposite way; we've found that we get better results if we start by studying the patient's lifestyle and eating habits, and then pattern the insulin regimen around that.

"I think that, traditionally, people viewed the dietitian as a person who limited choices and gave you a diet to follow. We were the food police who were going to take away your food. Today, however, I look at my role as being more of a patient advocate and empowerer. I show people how to manage food and maintain blood sugar control. It's a self-management approach."

Delahanty is not in the business of telling people what they can or cannot eat; she's more interested in helping them to understand what's behind food labels, which can often be misleading, and how to avoid surprises when ordering at restaurants, and how many calories are concealed in casseroles that may contain all kinds of foods.

"Many people still have that old image in mind," she says. "A doctor may tell the patient, 'You're not doing very well, you need to see a dietitian.' So it sounds like a punishment. In fact, the dietitian ought to be an integral part of the care, and that only happens when we empower the patient and help them to comply. We show them how to take charge."

To aid this process of education, Delahanty can offer four meal-planning approaches, each of which offers different features for different people. We'll learn more about those in Chapter 4.

Other Specialists

The other specialists on the team often come on the scene to screen for or prevent complications, or when a person with diabetes suffers from complications. People with diabetes need a specialist who both understands a particular disease or organ system *and* understands diabetes. Because diabetes can change your reaction to diseases and to medications, you may require a different treatment plan than would be used otherwise. There are a number of specialists whom you can expect to consult over the years.

If you are a woman with diabetes, pregnancy is a very serious matter; it brings a whole new meaning to the phrase "planned parenthood." Pregnancy is not something to leave to chance if you have diabetes, and you should start planning for it before trying to become pregnant. Chances are you'll need the services of an obstetrician schooled in diabetes care and management of "high-risk" pregnancy.

Everyone with diabetes should see an eye specialist regularly to monitor the onset of diabetic eye disease. An eye specialist, or ophthalmologist, can spot early signs of retinopathy, one of the most frequent complications of diabetes, and can help prevent this condition from worsening if it does arise. You should try to find an ophthalmologist who specializes in retinal diseases and sees patients with diabetes regularly. Your diabetologist can probably recommend someone.

Another frequent concern of people with diabetes is proper foot care. At Mass General, people who are at risk for foot problems or who already have them are frequently referred to a podiatrist for specialty care and procedures. Podiatrists undergo years of training, including instruction in the treatment of people with diabetes. Again, ask your diabetologist or primary care physician to recommend a podiatrist with experience in treating diabetes.

You may need to consult with specialists trained in the treatment of other serious diabetic conditions. Kidney disease, or nephropathy, is an all too common complication that is usually treated by a kidney specialist, or nephrologist. Diabetes, and especially NIDDM, is associated with abnormal levels of blood lipids, such as cholesterol, as well as high blood pressure and poor circulation, and many people with diabetes develop heart disease and blockage of circulation to the brain (stroke) and legs as a result. You may need to see a cardiologist to help you prevent or to treat heart disease and a vascular surgeon to relieve circulatory problems. Finally, a variety of nervous system complications (neuropathies) occur frequently in all forms of diabetes and may require help from a neurologist. A urologist may be needed to treat impotence or bladder problems.

There are many types of specialty health care personnel whom you may need to call on to cope with your diabetes. We often consult behavioral scientists (psychologists or psychiatrists) when patients are having difficulty adjusting to diabetes and its complications, or are not succeeding with their treatment regimen. The important thing to remember is that you need to find someone who is interested in treating people with diabetes, and who has the experience necessary to obtain the best possible outcome for you. Your diabetologist will often be able to take care of many of these problems and will hopefully know when additional input is required. Not all hospitals have as many diabetes specialists as Mass General, and you may have to look around to get the level of care you desire. Don't be afraid to ask questions, and pay close attention to how doctors, nurses, and other health care personnel treat you. Find out whether they treat significant numbers of patients with diabetes. Are they interested in your blood sugar levels and oral medication or insulin regimen? Do they make it their business to understand your goals for self-treatment? Can you talk to them freely and openly about problems, without feeling rushed, embarrassed, or demeaned? Do the specialists interact and communicate with your diabetes team? These are all important questions to consider when selecting a specialist. You don't have to follow your own doctor's referral; if you're not satisfied, discuss your dissatisfaction with him or her and keep looking. A good diabetes treatment team can help educate you, support you, and work with you to establish a self-treatment regimen that will keep you in good health for years to come.

4

Diet: Food for Life

"Do you eat to live? Or do you live to eat?" For just about all of us, I think, the answer is probably yes to both questions. Although we need to eat, we love to eat just as much. We need carbohydrates, proteins, fats, calories, vitamins, minerals, and all those other components you can read about on the side of a cereal box while you're trying to wake up. And if you don't get those nutrients in adequate amounts, you may put your health at risk. To hear some people talk, they would rather die than eat a calorie. And yet calories are anything but our enemies; they supply the energy you need to "get up and do what needs to be done," as humorist Garrison Keillor would say.

But the question of how much fat, protein, and carbohydrate should be in the diet—what amounts and in what form—is one that has been debated since the first diet book was published (probably only minutes after Gutenberg invented the printing press). Researchers are continually observing and experimenting with the human diet, looking for the most healthful way for people to eat. They are confounded, however, by several factors. One is the variety of human diets. Different cultures prepare and eat their foods in different ways. In the United States, there is really no one cultural diet; people live and eat in an almost infinite spectrum of microcultures, and many eat a wide variety of foods from day to day. The total number of calories and the amount of protein and fat derived from animal sources tends to be highest in wealthier, industrialized nations and lowest in the poorer, agrarian, developing countries. (Judging by the size of "average" portions in most U.S. restaurants and the large number of "all you can eat" restaurants, we are *by far* the wealthiest nation on earth.)

Although diets can be very predictable, there is another element that frustrates efforts to study them. This could be called "the human factor"—the principle that, no matter how many times you try to tell people what and how much they ought to eat, they inexorably and almost uniformly revert to eating habits that make them comfortable or suit their needs for the moment, despite the merit of whatever advice they've been given.

There's really nothing surprising in that. We've been brought up to enjoy our food. Most of us eat three times a day, and those three meals are probably the most consistent opportunities for pleasure and relaxation we get. Eating puts you in the driver's seat. It's a great feeling to eat what you want, when you want, as much as you want, as fast or as slow as you want. It's nice to eat with friends and take pleasure in their company whether dunking a donut or carving a roast duck. Holiday meals bring with them added excitement and anticipation: there are sights and smells and tastes to appreciate. A snack in the middle of a hard day's work is more than just nourishment—it's a reward.

The natural, perfectly understandable attachment people form to their eating habits has been a longtime obstacle to diabetes specialists. This "human factor" has interfered with naive attempts to impose rigid diets in free-living human beings. Careful control of diets in a real-life setting is problematic. Temptation is all around us.

But that hasn't stopped anyone from trying to define the "perfect" diet for people with diabetes. Before insulin became available in 1922, physicians and nutrition therapists devised many diets purported to extend the lives of, or even cure, people with diabetes. The most popular of these, the Allen diet, used at the beginning of the century, was an extremely low-carbohydrate, low-fat eating plan. This diet was intended to keep blood sugar as low as possible and to forestall the patient's inevitable descent into diabetic coma. Nevertheless, in most people, the long-term effects of living without insulin were bound to take their toll: muscle and fat cells starved. Patients slowly wasted away and eventually died of either infection, starvation, or the acute complications of diabetes, dehydration and acidosis.

After the lifesaving introduction of insulin, early researchers saw immediately that to use insulin to its full potential, patients needed to keep food intake, and especially carbohydrates, stable from day to day and meal to meal. The reason for this was simple: insulin *lowers* blood sugar levels, and food, especially the carbohydrate content, *raises* it. In order to keep blood sugar in a healthy range, you had to try to match food intake and insulin doses. During the first sixty years of insulin use, monitoring blood sugar was only performed in laboratories and wasn't available to patients. Gauging insulin needs using urine tests, which were widely used until the early 1980s, was nearly impossible.

Because it was so hard to determine blood sugar levels during daily activities before self–blood testing became available, diabetologists had to rely on less technological methods to try to help patients keep blood sugar levels in a healthy range. Physicians resorted to recommending highly consistent and restricted diets. These diets were aimed at keeping carbohydrate, protein, and fat content as constant as possible and distribute them during the day so that they would match the relatively unchanging insulin dose. When fat was recognized in the 1960s as a culprit in causing heart disease, it was also limited in diabetic diets. Protein was regarded as fairly neutral— necessary, but without grave consequences for the patient with diabetes.

To provide some flexibility for people with diabetes, "exchange" systems were developed. An exchange is a form of dietary currency. Each exchange is a unit of food, and an exchange within any of the principal food lists— starch, fruit, milk, vegetables, meat, and fats—has the same "worth" as any other exchange in that list. The major emphasis is on carbohydrate exchanges. Roughly speaking, that means that a slice of bread and a small (three-ounce) baked potato, which are both on the starch list, should have roughly the same nutritional value and impact on blood sugar, and they should be balanced, or "covered" by the same amount of insulin. Same for an ounce of Canadian bacon and an ounce of lean steak on the meat list, or a scoop of ice cream and an ounce of potato chips on the fats list. From your blood sugar's point of view, two food choices in the same list are "worth" about the same amount, and both are covered by about the same amount of insulin. (Of course, the amount of insulin required by an individual for one exchange can vary from person to person, depending on level of insulin resistance and other factors.) The exchange system made it possible to alter your diet (within defined limits) without altering your insulin dose, enabling you to maintain a relatively stable blood sugar. The exchange system was traditionally used to adjust food to match insulin.

"The exchange system was the first system people used to understand their diet, and it's not dead," says Linda Delahanty, R.D. In her role as a dietitian at Mass General, Linda helps people work with their diets to get maximum flexibility and acceptable blood sugar control simultaneously. "It continues to be useful as a means to achieve dietary consistency. But the exchange system isn't the only system. There are many meal-planning strategies that can be tailored to the person with diabetes. Some of these systems are simpler, and some are more flexible. This allows people with different lifestyles and dietary habits to achieve more success with them.

"It's not 'all or nothing,' especially with food," Delahanty says. "Diet is the hardest part of taking care of your diabetes, and it's very difficult to be perfect with your diet. But if you take care of 80 percent of your diet, it's going to make a big difference."

Linda was part of the research team involved in the Diabetes Control and Complications Trial (DCCT), a nationwide study of the relationship between blood sugar control and diabetes complications. An important part of the DCCT was to determine the best ways to facilitate tight blood sugar control. The development of methods for patients to measure blood glucose levels quickly, accurately, and relatively easily revolutionized diabetes care. Modern diabetes therapy takes advantage of blood glucose monitoring technology and the capability of adjusting insulin to match insulin to food, not vice versa.

"In the old days, when you developed diabetes, you

Eating Habits That Help Control Blood Sugar in IDDM

As part of Mass General's diabetes research team, and as a member of the team that carried out the Diabetes Control and Complications Trial, Linda Delahanty was interested in finding out how dietitians can help people with diabetes control their blood sugar. Linda's team found that there are some self-care habits that can help you control your blood sugar:

1. Stick to your meal plan. This can be hard to do, but as Linda says, try as hard as you can, and if you find that you *can't* stick to your meal plan, work with your dietitian to come up with a new plan that you *can* stick to.
2. Learn to adjust your insulin dosage according to what you plan to eat as well as according to blood glucose level and anticipated exercise. This takes time, and you will make some mistakes, but the effort is worth it. You'll feel much more confident and in control when you can make you own insulin decisions.
3. Treat insulin reactions promptly and appropriately. There's a common tendency to overtreat low blood sugars, and it's natural to do so, because no one wants their blood sugar to drop to the point where they can't treat themselves any longer. Appropriate self-treatment takes practice and patience. You must treat hypoglycemia as a medical emergency—the treatment is 4 to 6 ounces of orange juice or Coke, or a similar amount of rapidly available sucrose (table sugar). Don't use a

reaction as an excuse to eat anything and everything. Overtreatment only leads to elevated blood sugar. If you notice that insulin reactions tend to crop up at the same time of day consistently, talk to your diabetologist, your dietitian, or your diabetes educator right away. Together, you can determine why they are occurring and work out a solution.

4. Eat a consistent bedtime snack—and don't overdo it. Eating a bedtime snack can feel like a chore, especially if you wait until the last minute to take care of it. But without that bedtime snack you can leave yourself vulnerable to nighttime insulin reactions. On the other hand, some people try to protect themselves from nocturnal reactions with a heavy snack, and that can leave you with chronically elevated sugar through the night. Work with your treatment team to strike a happy medium, and then stick to it.

were given an insulin regimen and you were expected to work your diet around that," Delahanty says. "That was hard for a lot of people to do, because they were used to eating a certain way, and then we came along and told them, 'You can't eat the same way you've been eating all your life.' Basically, we were trying to mold habits around insulin. And although some people could make that adjustment, probably just as many couldn't, and many of them had poor results with their self-treatment.

"Now we've changed our approach. While we were preparing for and conducting the DCCT, we tried to find the best way to get people to make healthy food choices and adjust to their diet. We found that the best way was to start with their own lifestyle, their own eating habits, their own foods, and work from there. Now we pattern the insulin regimen around the eating habits and not the reverse.

And that seems to be more effective than the old approach."

A common example that demonstrates the difference between the older approach of adjusting the diet to match insulin and the modern approach of adjusting insulin to diet can be seen in the use of snacks. Older style diabetic diets often insisted on one snack between breakfast and lunch, and another between lunch and dinner. This was thought to be necessary to prevent the mid-morning and mid-afternoon hypoglycemia associated with the constant dose of insulin given in the morning. As Linda explains, the modern approach is different.

"For instance, a traditional diabetic diet would require you to eat an afternoon snack whether you were used to doing that or not. Well, your response *might* be to eat that afternoon snack, as you were told. On the other hand, your response *also* might be to forget about it, or postpone it until it was too late. Maybe it's the busiest time of the day where you work, and you try to do it, and sometimes you can and sometimes you can't. There are all kinds of possibilities, but the traditional approach would be to keep reminding you to eat that snack.

"Well, it would be a lot easier for both of us if we talked about the afternoon snack for a few minutes and about whether you thought you would be able to eat it. And maybe, if you said that it would be hard for you to manage, we might find another way of structuring your insulin dosage so that you wouldn't have to eat a snack at just that time. Rather than trying to fit your diet to the insulin, we try to fit your insulin regimen to your usual eating habits."

In other words, the modern approach is to determine whether you would like a snack at various times of the day and to decide whether or not to include that snack based on your overall caloric needs, exercise, work or school schedule, and other factors. If you don't want to snack at that time of day, your insulin dose can be adjusted with the help of results from blood sugar monitoring, so that your blood sugar will stay in a healthy range. This approach imitates what a normally functioning pancreas would do, matching insulin delivery to insulin needs.

It also makes sense. First of all, no doctor or dietitian can force someone to go on a diet he or she doesn't accept. As soon as you walk out of my office, you're very much on your own. If someone tries to take a diet and "ram it down your throat," you probably won't respond well. No one is going to stick with a diet just because they want to please me or Linda. You have to want to do it for yourself.

Gail Denman has been seeing Linda for advice about her diet. Because she had been treating her own diabetes since the age of nine, Gail felt that she "knew it all" when it came to diabetic nutrition and that her only problem was putting her knowledge into practice. Linda acknowledged that Gail had a handle on some dietary basics and knew the carbohydrate, fat, and protein content of many different foods. But what Linda tried to do was get Gail on a realistic diet that she could follow.

"I don't feel like a patient when I'm with Linda," Gail says. "I see us more as professionals working together."

Some of Gail's problems centered on her eating schedule. Her work with the Massachusetts Commission for the Blind involves visiting clients in their homes for teaching and counseling, and she frequently eats on the run. She asked Linda whether she could substitute a low-fat granola bar with yogurt and a piece of fruit for a sandwich at lunchtime. With monitoring to determine whether her choice of insulin dose for the substitution maintained acceptable sugar levels, Linda reassured Gail that she could try it.

"Linda also really wanted to focus on what I wanted to keep the same," Gail says. Her husband, Jim, was working late, not getting home for dinner until eight-thirty or nine-thirty in the evening. Gail was afraid that she would have to give up eating with Jim so that her blood sugars wouldn't bottom out before dinner.

"Linda recommended a few foods that I could have for a snack that wouldn't put me over the edge, and helped me adjust my insulin doses," Gail recalls. "She had some ideas that just made it a little healthier. I'm thrilled because my husband and I are still eating together."

Although this new philosophy of diabetes management is more realistic and flexible for many patients, it requires glucose monitoring and a good understanding of the effects of different foods on blood sugar control. For example, you can eat desserts in moderation, as long as you understand the need for adjusted insulin doses to maintain safe, acceptable glucose levels. Several years ago we investigated whether a previously forbidden food for diabetics, ice cream, could be safely incorporated into their diet. We discovered that with appropriate insulin coverage, moderate amounts of ice cream were safe (and delicious).

Now, does this mean that it's okay to hop into your car, drive to the ice cream stand, and have a double chocolate cone every night because you're covering it with insulin? Well, that depends on your dietary goals. If you have non-insulin-dependent diabetes, you know that there's a very good chance you can control your diabetes by losing weight. Good blood sugar control *can* reduce your risk of complications but *cannot* help you control your weight.

This is precisely the kind of thing that your dietitian will talk to you about in more detail. She or he will give you as much flexibility as possible while you try to take care of your blood sugar and your general health. And the more sugar and fat you eat, the harder that will be to do.

The other major goals of diets for IDDM and NIDDM are to help you achieve and maintain your ideal weight and decrease your risk for cardiovascular disease. These goals largely involve limitations of dietary fat, especially saturated fat and cholesterol, which further complicates a diabetic diet. If you have high blood pressure, which is very common in NIDDM, you may also need to restrict your sodium intake.

Some general nutritional guidelines that come from the American Dietetic Association's *Meal-Planning Approaches for Diabetes Management* are instructive. Eating healthy can sound unpleasant and unappealing at first. Then you realize that practically all professional athletes, many of your favorite entertainers, and many successful business people eat extremely healthy diets. They do so because it helps them perform at their best, and because they like the taste of "whole" healthy foods. And in some respects their healthy diets may be similar to the diet that we urge you to eat. It's not a "diabetic diet": it's a healthy diet, one that anyone who wants to feel good and live a long, healthy life ought to think about eating.

General Nutritional Guidelines

Fat

An important choice that many people can start making right away is to eat less fat. High dietary fat has been linked with both heart disease and cancer. People with diabetes are at elevated risk for heart disease and ought to try to avoid high-fat foods. In addition, high-fat foods are calorically dense, containing about twice as many calories as a similar volume of carbohydrate-rich food. Limiting high-fat foods is crucial for weight loss and weight control. Here are some ways to avoid high-fat foods:

• Eat less red meat and more fish and chicken. Red meat is loaded with fat, especially saturated fat, as well as cholesterol, both of which have been linked to heart disease.
• Avoid fried foods. Admittedly, fried foods are a way of life for many people. However, you can avoid eating lots of fat by broiling, baking, or roasting meat, and trimming fat and skin. If you have to eat something fried, sauté or stir-fry some zucchini rather than a half pound of bacon.
• Drink low-fat milk—1 percent, or better yet, skim.
• Other high-fat foods to limit include cheese, ice cream, and sour cream. Try the low-fat or fat-free versions, which get better all the time.

Incidentally, for those interested in vegetarian or vegan diets, the American Dietetic Association has taken the position that "vegetarian diets are healthful and nutritionally adequate" for people with diabetes, when appropriately planned. Keep in mind that any vegetarian diet is likely to be considerably higher in fiber and lower in fat than conventional eating patterns. So if you're considering vegetarianism, but are worried about the consequences, bring it up with your dietitian. You'll probably get an encouraging response. Substituting more salad, vegetables, and whole grains for high-fat foods is always desirable.

Fiber

Another important healthy habit that many people can cultivate is to eat more dietary fiber. Many nutritious, low-calorie foods are high in fiber, and you should get your daily share. Some of these high-fiber foods include:

- Whole fruit (not juice)
- Whole-grain breads and cereals
- Vegetables, green and otherwise
- Legumes, such as beans, peas, and lentils

Salt

In patients with high blood pressure, one of the first steps is to cut down on sodium consumption. You can easily do this at home, substituting other flavorings such as lemon, garlic, and other seasonings. What you *can't* change is how much salt fast food restaurants add to their food to make it more appetizing. So it's a good policy to avoid eating at fast-food restaurants and convenience stores.

Sugar

Let's talk about sugar, the diabetic's "enemy." In truth, we all need sugar in our diets. You need a source of sugar to survive—without it, you couldn't keep your blood sugar high enough to function.

So-called refined sugar does present some problems, however. In *Sugar Blues,* author William Dufty writes about the history of refined sugar, and the important role it played in the colonization of the New World. Sugar was prized as if it were gold in the late 1500s and early 1600s, and English sugarcane plantation owners in the West Indies bought slaves to provide the labor to make massive fortunes.

"The pleasure, glory and grandeur of England has been advanced more by sugar than any other commodity," said Sir Thomas Dalby in defense of the sugar trade. Indeed, contends Dufty, England had become "hooked" on refined sugar, and since that time, all of Western society has been hooked on it, too.

It's best to avoid large amounts of refined or simple sugars because of what they can do to your blood sugar level: rapidly send it sky-high. You can manage the impact of simple sugars or concentrated sweets, consumed in moderation, on blood sugar levels if you include them as part of your total carbohydrate for the meal or snack and know how to adjust your insulin doses; however, if you eat large amounts of concentrated sweets, it may be difficult to give yourself enough insulin to counteract the resulting rapid rise in blood sugar. For example, the sugar content of 12 ounces of soda or juice is so quickly digested and absorbed that it is difficult to match it with insulin.

Simple sugars can be found in table sugar, honey, syrup, jam, jelly, soft drinks, fruit juices, hard candy, and cake frosting, just to name a few foods. If you really like sweets, you may want to acquaint yourself with some sugar substitutes, such as saccharin, aspartame, and mannitol.

• Candy sweetened with sorbitol or mannitol has a kind of sweet, smoky taste that many patients like. The worst thing about it—and this is something I frequently hear from patients—is that it gives you intestinal gas, and even diarrhea if you eat a lot of it.

Will Life with Diabetes Still Be Sweet?

People who know nothing at all about the disease often assume that people with diabetes are allergic to sugar, are addicted to sugar, can't eat sugar under any circumstances, or caused their diabetes by eating too much sugar. *You* know that these things aren't true, but perhaps you like sweets. Over the years, it has been more or less axiomatic that people with diabetes should avoid the use of table sugar, or sucrose, at all costs, because of its tendency to raise blood sugar rapidly.

Whether people with diabetes ought to avoid sugar *completely* has come into question. New guidelines from the American Diabetes Association state that "sucrose [table sugar] as part of the meal plan does not impair blood glucose control in individuals with type I [IDDM] or type II [NIDDM] diabetes. Sucrose and other sucrose-containing foods must be substituted for other carbohydrates and foods and not simply added to the meal plan. In making such substitutions, the nutrient content of concentrated sweets . . . must be considered."

What this means is that there is no reason for you to avoid sweets completely, *as long as they are accounted for in your meal plan.* If and when you eat sweets, you must take them into account with regard to total carbohydrates and total calories, and make sure that the sweets that you do eat are covered with insulin (we'll learn more about insulin coverage in Chapter 5). One of the advantages of the new treatment philosophy of matching insulin delivery to insulin need is that it allows you greater dietary flexibility. As long as you give yourself enough insulin, appropriately timed, to match your intake, sweets can be a part of your diet. Of course, the major issue in NIDDM is the control of total calories. To the extent that sweets sabotage most weight-loss diets, avoid or limit them.

"People used to think of the dietitian as the person who took food away from them," says dietitian Linda Delahanty.

(continued)

Will Life with Diabetes Still Be Sweet? *(cont'd)*

"That's *not* what we do. We try to help you find a way to eat the foods you're used to eating—even if that means eating the occasional candy bar—and to keep your blood sugar under control at the same time. You may have to make some compromises, but we can almost always work something out."

This is very good news for people with a sweet tooth, but remember—*this does not mean that you can throw your meal plan away and eat sweets.* On the contrary, you ought to consult closely with your diabetes treatment team, and particularly with your dietitian, to find out how to include your favorite sweets in your diet.

• Saccharin is the sweetener found in Sweet'n Low. Tab, one of the first popular diet soft drinks, is sweetened with saccharin. Many people lost their taste for saccharin when experiments with laboratory animals hinted that it may cause cancer. However, the animals in these experiments were fed saccharin in amounts that, in humans, would equal more than a hundred bottles of soft drink per day. Also, as is often said in scientific circles, a rat is not a human being. So, many people continue to use saccharin without worry.

• Aspartame is another name for NutraSweet, a more recently developed sweetener, also used to sweeten diet soft drinks. For a variety of reasons, the world has taken aspartame-sweetened diet soft drinks to heart, and you can find it in Diet Pepsi, Diet Coke, Diet Sprite, and all sorts of other drinks. Aspartame has been associated with certain birth defects of the nervous system called neural tube defects (for example, spina bifida). There have also been some reports of an association with pancreatic cancer. Again, these associations have been made in experiments with laboratory animals treated with huge doses. There is no evidence that aspartame causes problems in humans.

Sucrose is the sugar in table sugar; it has two molecules of glucose that are released with digestion. Fructose is the predominant sugar found in fruits. Remember that there is very little difference between fructose and sucrose in their ability to raise your blood sugar. Fructose is slightly more complex than refined sugar, so it takes a little longer to break down; therefore, it won't cause your blood sugar to rise quite as precipitously. However, make sure that anyone who cooks for you knows that fructose is *not* sugar free. (You can buy fructose for cooking in the grocery store.)

Don't automatically think that food labeled "low fat" and "all natural" can be eaten without consequences. Low-fat foods can be very high in carbohydrates and can raise your blood sugar to a very high level. "Diet" food can be very high in fat, and that's something you ought to be careful of, for reasons we outlined above. Learn to read labels. "All-natural" foods are frequently high in sugar and fat. "Sugar free" seldom means that a food is calorie free. If you do try a new snack food, make sure you read the label, and get a good idea of how many calories, fat, and sugar you're consuming. See the sidebar on food labels.

The ADA guidelines are by no means a precise guide to diabetic nutrition, but they are a good place to start. Anyone can use these guidelines, whether you're a Ph.D. or a first-grader. But if you want to control your blood sugar and have more freedom with your diet, you'll need to look at some dietary planning options that require a little thinking on your part.

Many persons with diabetes develop an innate sense of

Read It and Eat: New Food Labeling Guidelines

How many times have you stared at the side of a food box, trying vainly to figure out exactly what is in it, and knowing that you're at the mercy of the people who wrote the label?

In 1993, under pressure from the American Diabetes Association, the American Dietetic Association, and other groups, the federal Food and Drug Administration approved new, strict food-labeling guidelines that closely regulate what manufacturers can say about their food, and how they can say it. From now on, the words *low fat* will actually mean something when they appear on the outside of a cereal box. And you will find very detailed information about the food's nutritional content on the label outside, in a form that we hope you will be able to decipher easily.

The front panel of a box or can of food is much more closely regulated than ever before. "Sugar free" now means something very specific: less than half a gram of sugar per serving. A food that is labeled either "light" or "lite" must have one third fewer calories or 50 percent less fat per serving than the "non-light" food from which it takes its name. A "light" cream cheese, for example, must have one third the calories or half the fat of "regular" cream cheese. "Fat free" means that the food has less than one-half gram per serving. A complete list of the new definitions can be obtained from the American Diabetes Association.

The nutritional information label has also been changed to make understanding easier. First, serving sizes have been standardized between manufacturers, to make comparisons between similar foods easier. The label then tells you how many calories are in each serving, and the number of grams and percentages of fat, cholesterol, sodium, carbohydrate, and protein each serving contains. The amount of carbohydrate from dietary fiber and sugars are also listed. Sugars include all sucrose, fructose, maltose, lactose, brown sugar, high fructose corn syrup, and fruit juice concentrate. Of course, nothing on the label magically prevents you from overeating—unless you glue the label over your lips. Six servings of a "light" dessert at a single sitting will add up to a lot of fat and calories. For the most part, you must still exercise a degree of old-fashioned self-control.

the impact that specific groupings of food, better known as meals, will have on their blood sugar. Based on this sense, they become adept at choosing insulin doses to match specific meals. Unfortunately, this approach is limited and many patients don't develop this ability. To help her in accommodating different patients' needs, dietitian Linda Delahanty uses several different meal-planning guides, each designed for different types of patients with different abilities and needs for controlling their diets. Some of these approaches are applied most often in IDDM. In NIDDM, limiting the total number of calories and total fat is usually more important than the specific distribution of calories throughout the day. However, patients with NIDDM may find that these approaches help them organize their dieting efforts (see Chapter 10 for further discussion of diet and NIDDM).

Although the systems vary in their complexity and approach to meal planning, most patients can use at least one of these approaches successfully. There is no right or wrong system, no better or worse. However, some of these approaches are more suited for beginners and others for experienced "pros." They are provided to give people with diabetes choices in managing their diets. Here are some of the different approaches:

• Individual guidelines. A set of two to four personal goals that you and your dietitian agree will help improve your blood sugar control. For example, limit the size or frequency of snacks.

• Sample menus. Personalized sample menus that take into account your food preferences and eating habits.

• Healthy Food Choices. The simplest food-planning system to use, and a starting point for learning the exchange system for many newly diagnosed diabetics.

- The Exchange System. Over the years, probably the most widely used system. Exchanges are usually single serving amounts of food that can help make calculation of your calorie intake easier.
- Carbohydrate Counting System. A more flexible system that requires people to count carbohydrates in their diet. Using this information, they can better understand the impact of foods on blood sugar and decide how much insulin coverage they need.

Let's examine them in detail.

Individual Guidelines

Linda Delahanty told me about a young high school boy who had trouble following a diet. "He didn't do much with his diabetes, and he had a lot of high and low readings. He was testing occasionally but not much—he just wasn't really with the program. Like a lot of young people, he ate in an erratic fashion, slept late whenever he could, and might skip breakfast—even lunch."

When Linda noticed that her young patient had no systematic pattern of eating, she became concerned. He was free of medical problems for the time being, she knew, except for some daily high and low blood sugars that made him feel "rotten." But if this were allowed to continue, it could lead to serious diabetic complications down the road. This boy had to start thinking about diabetes in a very concrete way, to set some basic dietary goals and try to stick to them: an initial goal might be to try to eat three meals every day. The only way that a patient at this level of coping with diabetes could progress was with very small steps, one at a time.

Healthy Food Choices is a simplified version of the exchange system and is the most basic of the diabetic meal plans. It's a simple plan: you can use Healthy Food Choices without being meticulous about measuring your food, and you don't have to count calories. You only have to count the few food choices that you make each day.

Here's how it works. Every day, whether you think about it or not, you choose what to eat—one glass of milk, an apple, a sandwich, spaghetti, and so on. Each of these choices is part of your overall diet for that day. The Healthy Food Choices system adds a little extra meaning to the word *choices;* each choice is a standard amount of food in one of six categories: starch, vegetables, milk, meat and fish, fruit, and fat. All choices in the same category are roughly equivalent in their caloric value. For example, half a cup of pasta equals one starch choice, as does one third of a cup of rice, as does half an English muffin (see "Healthy Food Choices" on pages 76–77).

If you haven't been monitoring your own diet for very long, you probably can't think in exact terms about how much you're eating. But as you go along, you'll learn to "size up" your food, even in restaurants, which usually pose the greatest challenge. For instance, if you estimate that you've eaten two cups of pasta at one sitting, that's four ½-cup choices.

After taking a diet history and reviewing your insulin dosage, your dietitian will work with you to establish how many choices you will make from each category for each meal and snack. For instance, you may decide that for dinner, you'll make two starch choices, four meat, two fat, one vegetable, one fruit, and one milk. After a while, you may find that you're more comfortable eating three starches, but two fats are too many for you. Your treat-

Healthy Food Choices

Each day you need to eat a variety of foods. Each person's daily calorie and nutritional needs are different. A nutrition counselor can help you work out how many choices from each food group are just right for you. By eating foods from each food group, you will meet your basic nutritional needs. For a healthy diet, each day you should have at least 4 choices from the starch/bread group; 5 meat or meat substitute choices; 2 vegetable choices; 2 fruit choices; 2 skim milk choices; and not more than 3 fat choices. These choices add up to about 1200 calories per day.

The foods listed in each group are just examples. Many others can be part of your daily meal plan.

STARCH/BREAD

Each of these equals one starch/bread choice (80 calories)

You have____choices each day.

1/2 cup pasta or barley
1/3 cup rice or cooked dried
   beans and peas
1 small potato (or 1/2 cup mashed)
1/2 cup starchy vegetables
   (corn, peas, or winter squash)
1 slice bread or 1 roll

1/2 English muffin, bagel, or
   hamburger/hot dog bun
1/2 cup cooked cereal
3/4 cup dry cereal, unsweetened
4–6 crackers
3 cups popcorn, unbuttered, not
   cooked in oil

MEAT AND SUBSTITUTES

You have____choices each day.

Each of these equals one meat choice (75 calories)

1 oz. cooked poultry, fish, or meat
1/4 cup cottage cheese
1/4 cup salmon or tuna, water packed
1 Tbsp. peanut butter
1 egg (limit to 3 per week)
1 oz. low-fat cheese, such as Mozzarella, ricotta

Each of these equals two meat choices (150 calories)

1 small chicken leg or thigh
1/2 cup cottage cheese or tuna

Each of these equals three meat choices (225 calories)

1 small pork chop
1 small hamburger
cooked meat, about the size of a deck of cards
1/2 of a whole chicken breast
1 medium fish fillet

VEGETABLES
Each of these equals one vegetable choice (25 calories)
You have_____choices each day.

1/2 cup cooked vegetables
1 cup raw vegetables
1/2 cup tomato/vegetable juice

FRUIT
Each of these equals one fruit choice (60 calories)
You have_____choices each day.

1 fresh medium fruit
1 cup berries or melon
1/2 cup canned in juice or without sugar
1/2 cup fruit juice
1/4 cup dried fruit

MILK
Each of these equals one milk choice.
The calories vary for each choice.
You have_____choices each day.

1 cup skim milk (90 calories)
1 cup lowfat milk (120 calories)
8-ounce carton plain lowfat yogurt (120 calories)

FAT
Each of these equals one fat choice (45 calories)
You have_____choices each day.

1 teaspoon margarine, oil, mayonnaise
2 teaspoons diet margarine or diet mayonnaise
1 tablespoon salad dressing
2 tablespoons reduced-calorie salad dressing

ment team will work with you to decide how to adjust your insulin and exercise regimen to compensate for the change. Perhaps you'll find out that, although these choices work all right for you during the week, you're eating more over the weekend. Again, discuss these adjustments with your treatment team, and get their advice. When you begin making Healthy Food Choices, it's a good idea to keep a detailed history of your diet and blood sugars to see how you're adjusting.

The Exchange System

The Exchange System was developed in 1950 by the American Diabetes Association and the American Dietetic Association to give some consistency but accommodate increased breadth to diabetic meal planning. It has been modified several times (most recently in 1995) and is the most established and probably the most widely used diabetes nutrition system today.

The word *exchange* has a meaning similar to that of the choices in the Healthy Food Choices system. Each exchange is interchangeable with other exchanges in the same category. The most recent revision divides food into three main groups: carbohydrate, meat, and fat. The carbohydrate group offers the flexibility to interchange fruit, starch, and milk choices. You and your dietitian will decide how many exchanges from each category to eat at each meal. In this way, you "set" your level of carbohydrate intake, so that you can choose the right amount of regular insulin to keep your blood sugar levels in the target range. It won't work perfectly at first, but you can work with your treatment team to adjust your insulin to your diet and exercise patterns.

The major difference between the Exchange System and Healthy Food Choices is that the Exchange System is much more precise, defining foods in terms of grams of carbohydrate, fat, and protein. This gives you a much clearer idea of how certain foods will affect your blood sugar and how much insulin you ought to be taking to cover them. Another major difference is that the Exchange System includes a much wider variety of foods. If you decide to use the Exchange System, you will use a copy of the book *Exchange Lists for Meal Planning* to determine the nutritional content of your food.

The Exchange System sounds complicated, but, in fact, children have been using this system for years to learn how to plan their meals. Kids seem to pick it up fairly easily. But adults can learn the exchange system, too. One of my patients, who was diagnosed at age twenty-eight, says it took about five days to get the hang of the Exchange System. She bought a scale and measuring cups so that she could make sure that her estimates of portion sizes were correct. Now it's second nature to her; she seldom consults a book or scale, she just estimates how much she's going to eat and then tries to stick close to her estimate when she sits down to the table. She still likes to measure everything very carefully when she cooks from a recipe: it gives her confidence to know exactly how much flour, sugar, and other ingredients are going into her food. As you'll see, this kind of information can be very important to controlling your blood sugar in the prescribed range.

Becoming acquainted with the Exchange System is an interesting process, because you learn much more about food than most people know: how many calories are in an eight-ounce steak, for instance, or how much fat is in peanut butter. It's this kind of information that is well worth knowing (and not just for people with diabetes). The Exchange System also tells you about relatively high-fiber, low-calorie food ("free foods"), such as pickles, raw vegetables, and butterless popcorn.

The Exchange System allows you to take more control of your diet, and it gives you confidence. You're no longer worrying about highs and lows, and reacting to them when they occur; you're in the driver's seat, keeping your sugar in control.

Carbohydrate Counting

Carbohydrate ("carbo") counting represents a slightly different and slightly more flexible approach to dietary management. The emphasis is not on which foods and how much, but on the potential each food has to alter blood sugar. When using the Healthy Food Choices and Exchange System approaches, your count is based on the amount of each food that you eat. In carbohydrate counting, you add up the amount of carbohydrate you eat at each meal and snack in order to predict how your blood sugar level will react. One way to look at it is that, rather than buying gas for your car by the tankful, you decide to pay for it by counting the units of octane that actually power your car.

Another fundamental difference is that carbohydrate counting, once you put in a little more work, is designed to give you more flexibility in what you eat. This system helps you "set" your carbohydrate intake so that it's consistent from day to day. This way, your insulin dose doesn't need much adjusting to accommodate different meals, since most meals will have a similar amount of carbohydrate if you stick to your diet plan.

Carbohydrate counting will allow you and your treatment team to determine how much glucose your body will make out of the food you eat. Then you can work out with them a range of insulin doses needed to cover your usual carbohydrate intake. Carbohydrate counting does take more thought and planning, but for many people it's worth it. This method is probably the most useful for people who are taking four shots a day, one before each meal (see Chapter 11 for discussion about intensive therapy). You don't have to be on intensive therapy to make use of this system; it will help you adjust your insulin dose to accommodate changes in diet no matter how many injections you take.

There are three levels of carbohydrate counting to learn. The first level focuses on learning how to count carbohydrates in meals and snacks and encourages you to eat similar amounts of carbohydrates from breakfast to breakfast, lunch to lunch, et cetera. The second level teaches you to observe how your blood sugar reacts to various amounts of carbohydrate. During this introductory period, you should try to keep your eating schedule as regular and consistent as possible. That way you will get a clearer sense of how your blood sugar responds to different carbohydrates and selected doses of insulin, without the added variability of changing mealtimes. The third level teaches you how to adjust your insulin doses based not only on your blood sugar level, but on the amount of carbohydrate in a specific meal.

This last level is most often used in intensively treated IDDM patients, but is useful for anyone who adjusts rapid-acting insulin before meals. For example, for every 10 to 15 grams of extra carbohydrate, you might need 1 additional unit of rapid-acting insulin. So suppose you were getting ready to eat your usual breakfast of 6 ounces of orange juice, a slice of toast, and a nectarine, totaling about 50 grams of carbohydrate and requiring about 4 units of rapid-acting insulin. If you decided to add a second slice of toast (15 grams of carbohydrate), you would probably add an extra unit of rapid-acting insulin for a total of 5 units. Of course, you would also adjust the dose depending on your blood sugar level before the meal. With the help of your diabetes treatment team, you should be fine-tuning your insulin dosage within a couple of weeks and can then incorporate variations in scheduling of meals.

So there you are. Take your pick from these meal-planning approaches. Or if you want to hear about other approaches to diabetic diet management, simply make an appointment with your diabetic treatment team. Remember, the point is not to fit you into the diet; it's to make the diet guidelines fit you—your work schedule, your sleep habits, your lifestyle, your exercise level, your appetite. You're never going to be able to control your blood sugar until you gain an understanding and at least a modicum of control over what you're eating, so make the decision to do it right away.

5

Insulin:
An Owner's Manual

The discovery of insulin is a story of brilliance, courage, stupidity, tenacity, insight, foolishness, greed, selflessness, inspiration, suffering, heroism, and, perhaps most of all, luck. Despite this somewhat inauspicious start, the discovery of insulin has proved to be one of the most beneficial in the annals of medicine. Unfortunately, the history of insulin's discovery is too long and involved for synopsis here; anyone interested in this exciting story can read the excellent book *The Discovery of Insulin,* by the Canadian historian Michael Bliss.

How Insulin Works

If your hormones were organized into a corporation, insulin would certainly be the treasurer. Insulin's function is to promote uptake and storage of glucose (sugar) and other nutrients. As such, insulin is one of the major anabolic or growth-promoting hormones. Some organs can use sugar and fatty acids, derived from fat, as an energy source, while the brain, the kidneys, and red blood cells use only sugar. Insulin ensures that glucose levels are regulated so that there is an adequate amount to satisfy the body's requirements under all conditions, including fasting, after eating, and during strenuous exercise. The amount of insulin secreted from the pancreas under these different conditions varies, with the major signal being the glucose level itself.

"Glucose and insulin are locked in a tightly interactive system," says Dr. Joseph Avruch, a Mass General researcher. "When blood sugar goes up, insulin goes up *immediately* and pushes the blood sugar level back down. As blood sugar levels fall, the stimulus to secrete insulin is withdrawn. When the level of insulin goes down, blood sugar bobs back up again. These two levels are constantly waxing and waning, regulating each other with feedback. The ultimate result is maintenance of stable glucose levels to supply the cells that need it in order to function properly."

Insulin controls blood sugar levels and helps supply it to the organs that depend on it in several ways. In order for glucose to be carried optimally into cells, molecules on the cell surface called *glucose transporters* must bind to the glucose and carry it from the bloodstream into the cells. Once the sugar is internalized, it must be broken down to provide energy. Neither of these processes occurs normally in the absence of appropriate insulin levels. The transport of sugar into the cells is blocked and the sugar that gets into the cells isn't used properly. In addition, the liver can be an organ of glucose uptake and storage or a source of glucose production. When insulin levels are high, the liver absorbs and stores glucose; when insulin levels are low, the liver releases glucose into the circulation. Therefore, when insulin levels are abnormally low, these effects lead to a large increase in blood sugar levels because of decreased storage of sugar by muscle, fat, and the liver, and increased sugar output by the liver (see the figure below). Even though the level of sugar in blood is high, the cells cannot use it; they are essentially starving for nutrition. On the other hand, when insulin levels are normally elevated, for example after a meal, sugar is stored in muscle cells, fat cells, and those of the liver (see the figure on p. 86). In the setting of inappropriately high insulin levels—for example, when an insulin-treated patient injects too much insulin—blood sugar concentrations fall to an abnormally low level as glucose is pushed into muscle, fat, and the liver, and the secretion of sugar from

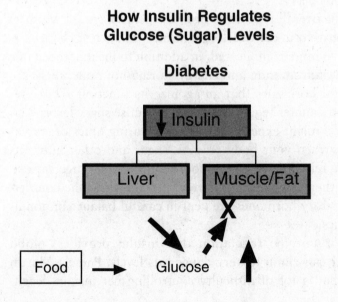

How Insulin Regulates
Glucose (Sugar) Levels

Diabetes

How Insulin Regulates
Glucose (Sugar) Levels

After a Meal

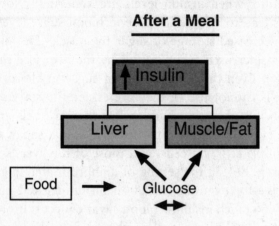

the liver ceases. The resulting low blood sugar, or hypo-glycemia, can be dangerous (see the figure on p. 87 and chapter 7).

The overall regulation of body *metabolism*—a wonderful term from the Greek that means "to alter or change"—is even more complicated. In addition to insulin, the major growth-promoting and energy-storing hormone, there are several hormones that antagonize its function. These so-called counter-regulatory hormones raise sugar levels, and as you might expect, they increase during times of starvation, when your body requires sugar and other nutrients to be released into the bloodstream from storage sites so that they can be used for energy. Insulin and the counter-regulatory hormones are kept in careful balance in nondiabetics.

Without the regulation that insulin provides, blood sugar can climb to very dangerous levels. Pamela Martin has had a lot of difficulty controlling her insulin-depen-

How Insulin Regulates
Glucose (Sugar) Levels

Hypoglycemia

dent diabetes for many years and has lost much of her vision and kidney function. Before she received a kidney transplant, Pamela underwent several years of dialysis treatment. Although this treatment was necessary for her survival, it caused large swings in her blood sugar. While showering one day, Pamela suffered a seizure from *high* blood sugar—a fairly rare occurrence, even among people with diabetes. Had her boyfriend Kurt not been there, she might not be alive today.

"I remember it coming on as it was happening to me because it felt like a rush went through my body," Pamela recalls. "It started in my feet and crept up. I called to Kurt because I could feel something was happening, and it just happened so quickly. I said, 'Kurt,' and that was it. The lights went out, and that's all I remember."

Blood sugars high enough to cause this kind of seizure

are very rare. For most people, the threat of high blood sugar lies in chronic high levels that lead to complications. As you probably already know, and will read more about later in this book, the long-term complications of diabetes continue to afflict many people, despite the high quality of care we have available for diabetics today. Vision impairment, kidney disease and failure, painful nervous system complications, amputations, heart disease, and other related health problems can be prevented with daily attention to your diabetic regimen.

The First Step—Monitoring

People who treat their diabetes successfully become very good observers. They are vigilant and respond rapidly by adjusting their insulin if changes in their diet, exercise, or daily schedule affect their blood sugar levels. In a sense, a person with IDDM learns to behave like her pancreas would, if it were functioning normally.

Unfortunately, your blood sugar control is no longer automatic. Blood sugar patterns, the causes for variations, and your responses need to be observed and recorded. When blood sugar is abnormally high or low, you don't just shake your head and wonder, you treat it and look for an explanation so that you can prevent a recurrence.

To become a "good pancreas," you need to start by observing and keeping a careful record of monitoring. Use a notebook to write down your blood sugars every day. This is one of the first things that Mass General diabetes educator Kathy Hurxthal asks people with diabetes to do. The notebook ought to be small enough to fit into your pocket, purse, or monitor pack. Each time you monitor, record the date and time that you tested your blood sugar, and the value. Useful diaries are often provided free of charge by the companies that manufacture diabetes treatment supplies. Remember, there's no point in writing down higher or lower numbers than you actually have, or in making up a blood sugar level if you didn't actually monitor. It won't impress your doctor, and it won't help you. If you're disappointed with your blood sugars, pretend that you're a newspaper reporter, and these are someone else's blood sugar numbers you are writing down. "Just the facts, ma'am" should be your motto.

Kathy further advises: "Try to monitor at consistent times, preferably before meals. As you learn more about how your body responds to food and exercise, you can begin to adjust your insulin dose to match those changes. This will keep your blood sugar in better control and give you more freedom to eat and exercise at your own convenience."

As you go on monitoring and recording your blood sugars, insulin doses, and changes in diet and exercise, you will quickly see patterns in your diabetes. What does your blood sugar do when you have a turkey sandwich, as opposed to vegetarian pizza? How does a bowl of Kix compare with Cheerios? How much more insulin do you need if your breakfast includes ice cream? What happens when you bike to work instead of taking the subway? And so on.

Some monitors make it easier for you by automatically storing your results. Several monitors have the capability to store multiple blood sugar readings, which can then be transferred to a computer for charting and analysis. However, to the extent that these "convenient" meters stop you from frequently recording blood sugars and the pertinent details of daily living that keep you tuned into your blood sugar patterns, they may actually interfere with good self-care. Keeping an up-to-date record in a timely fashion—in other words, as it happens—is critical.

Which Insulin, How Much and When

Before you had diabetes, your pancreas dutifully provided all the insulin you needed to keep your blood sugar in a healthy range. It probably seldom went above 120 mg/dl, even after a rich meal, or below 60 mg/dl. (Although there is a slow but steady increase in blood sugar levels that comes with aging, values don't normally exceed 120 fasting or 200 mg/dl after meals.) This exquisite control was due to the coordinated release of insulin and other hormones in response to diet, exercise, and blood sugar level, a system that has evolved to near perfection.

Now, your body's capacity to regulate blood sugar on its own has departed, leaving you with the responsibility. Until now, you never had to think about how much insulin it took to keep your blood sugar in a specified range. Your body made all the decisions for you and did it well enough so that you never had to get involved. With diabetes, the period of "automatic" insulin dosage is over. It's as though you had to put your calculator down and go back to calculating by hand. It's not easy. You would have a very tough time convincing me to turn off my word processor and revert to a pen and paper; even a typewriter seems to be a real inconvenience. So when you find out that you have diabetes and have to switch from an automatic insulin system to a "manual" one, it can be discouraging.

Still, it can be done. You can regulate your blood sugars

extremely well, perhaps better than you have ever imagined, if you pay attention to the principal factors of diet, exercise monitoring, and insulin. Of these, insulin is probably the hardest for most people to understand, at least at first. But that understanding can come quickly. People who use insulin and pay close attention to the effects it has on their glucose levels soon find themselves experimenting with different dosages and adjusting the times of their injections to accommodate diet and lifestyle decisions. Some people with IDDM take the step of using insulin pumps that in some ways mimic the function of the pancreas. Some people with NIDDM may find that with strict attention to diet and exercise, they can control their blood sugar without the use of insulin or oral medications. Both of these approaches take great dedication and attention to detail. Yet what they give in return is the promise of better health and more personal freedom.

It's important to remember that once your doctor prescribes insulin treatment, you can't take it intermittently, or forget it for a few days. If you have insulin-dependent diabetes, you depend totally on the insulin you take; skipping an insulin dose will result in a rapid increase in blood sugar levels; missing your doses for a few days will lead to dehydration, a breakdown of fat, resulting in a buildup of acid in the blood (ketoacidosis), and even death if not treated aggressively. (There's a full description of how ketoacidosis, or DKA, occurs in Chapter 1.) One of the major causes of DKA is that people with IDDM, who know they need insulin, stop taking it, either because they can't afford it, can't get access to it, or think they can go a few days without it. Sometimes people decrease or stop their dose when they have a flu and lose their appetite. While insulin may need adjustment in this circumstance, it should never be stopped. Remember: Your body needs insulin every day, and if your pancreas isn't producing it, you are responsible for injecting it every day, or you are headed for trouble. If you find it difficult to get the insulin you need, contact your doctor, nurse, or social worker and make sure he or she understands your problem. If you have NIDDM, stopping insulin usually won't cause DKA; however, it can lead to very high levels of blood sugar and make you feel pretty sick.

Types of Insulin

The main difference between the various types of insulin has to do with how rapidly they begin to act and the length of time they remain active after injection (see the figure on p. 95). All insulins are injected subcutaneously, under the most superficial layer of skin and into the fat layer below. Almost any area with a fat layer that you can reach, including the abdomen, hips, thighs, and the back of your upper arms, can be used for injection sites. Although parents often help very young children with their injections, we encourage everyone else to self-inject. Being independent not only frees you from relying on others, but will make you feel more confident about your diabetes care.

The syringes available today come in a variety of sizes, depending on how much insulin you inject. They all have extremely sharp needles that are almost entirely painless, resulting in a small "sting" at most. Almost everyone to whom we teach self-injection is initially hesitant about "doing it." However, within several days to weeks, the vast majority of insulin-injecting patients are very comfortable and wonder in retrospect what the fuss was all about.

The main varieties of insulin are the following:

Rapid-Acting Insulin

These insulins have a relatively rapid onset of activity (see the figure on p. 95), thus bringing blood sugar levels down quickly. Rapid-acting insulin—usually called *regular* or *clear*, because of its appearance—is normally taken before a meal to cope with the influx of glucose that occurs. The goal is to mimic the high level of insulin your pancreas would supply in response to an abrupt, high blood sugar level.

Rapid-acting insulin begins lowering your blood sugar about half an hour after injection; therefore, you should try to take your regular insulin half an hour *before* eating. Some people with IDDM discover that they need to take it even earlier—forty-five to sixty minutes before a meal—to achieve satisfactory control. Insulin action reaches its maximum level of blood sugar lowering activity about two hours after injection. Coincidentally, this is about the same time that your digestive processes are releasing the highest amount of sugar into your bloodstream from your meal.

Timing insulin injections appropriately before meals is sometimes difficult. My coauthor, John Lauerman, told me that his wife Judi and her college friends were once heading out to celebrate the end of exams with a small dinner, and she thought it would be best to inject her insulin on the way there. When they arrived at the restaurant, there was a long line to get in, and Judi's insulin was beginning to work. Judi was able to let someone know she needed someting to eat, but she ended up getting a little hypoglycemic anyway.

Remember to make sure that food will be available soon after you take your insulin. This may be difficult when you eat out. If the main course or appetizers are delayed in a restaurant, and you have already injected your rapid-acting insulin, you may need to ask for a glass of juice to sip while you wait. Don't worry, most restaurants are used to helping people with diabetes.

Rapid-acting insulins are usually active for four to as long as eight hours after injection. The larger the dose, the longer the duration. Unfortunately, the relatively long duration of rapid-acting insulin does not imitate the insulin pattern that occurs after a meal in non-diabetic people. In non-diabetics, insulin levels rise and fall very rapidly, so that the insulin level two to three hours after a meal has returned to the low level it was before the meal. On the other hand, rapid-acting insulin remains at a relatively higher level for as long as four to eight hours after injection. This rather long "tail" on its action profile can cause hypoglycemia if the next meal is delayed (see the figure on p. 95). To address this problem a new very rapid-acting insulin called Humalog has been developed. This insulin has a quicker onset and a shorter duration of action. This profile of activity will eliminate the need to inject quite as far in advance of the meal as is currently required, and should decrease the risk for hypoglycemia. This new insulin should be more convenient, especially for IDDM patients using frequent injections.

Intermediate Insulins

NPH (Neutral Protamine Hagedorn) and lente insulins take longer to begin lowering blood sugar levels, peak later, and have longer durations than rapid-acting insulins (see the figure opposite). All slower-acting insulins are cloudy in appearance (unlike the clear, short-acting insulin solutions) and they are designed to provide a more steady level of insulin than regular insulin.

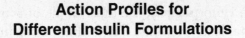

Action Profiles for Different Insulin Formulations

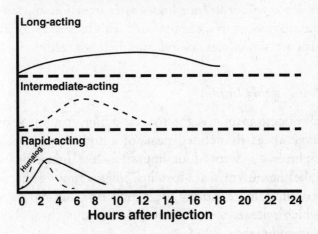

Protamine is a protein that is added to insulin to slow its absorption from the injection site and Hagedorn is the name of the person who developed this insulin. Lente (from the Latin word for slow) insulin works more slowly because of the addition of zinc. When it's time for an injection of NPH or lente, roll the container back and forth between your hands momentarily before filling the syringe. This ensures that there is equal distribution of the insulin throughout the fluid you are injecting.

NPH and lente insulins both begin to work one to two hours after injection, peak four to eight hours later, and last from eight to twelve hours. If you take NPH or lente in the morning, it should cover you for lunch and the afternoon, so it's important to inject at a regular time and eat at the right time, too, in order to avoid hypo- or hyperglycemia. If you take a dose of NPH or lente before bedtime, you are not depending on it to cover a meal; its purpose is to keep your blood sugar in control throughout the night. Unfortunately, the time profile of action is not as predictable as we would like to think. Sometimes NPH or lente will peak four hours after injection and on other days it may peak six hours later. This lack of absolute consistency sometimes complicates diabetes care.

Long-acting Insulin

Ultralente insulin is the longest-acting insulin; it doesn't have an easily defined peak of activity and lasts about eighteen to twenty-four hours (see the figure on p. 95). Like the intermediate insulins, long-acting insulin is used to mimic more closely the action of a normal pancreas, which releases a small amount of insulin throughout the day and night.

Premixed Insulins

There are several types of premixed insulins that provide a mixture of rapid- and intermediate-acting insulins in a fixed ratio. One commonly used premixed insulin, called "70/30," gives a premixed dose of 70 percent NPH insulin and 30 percent regular insulin. The good thing about a premixed insulin is that you can use one injection to cover much of your day. We'll talk about this in the next section, too.

By the way, you can also mix your own insulins, if need be and with your doctor's approval. Mixing your own insulins allows you to customize your injections. For example, before a particularly large breakfast you may want to mix a large dose of regular insulin with your usual NPH dose. Always make sure that you draw up the regular insulin first and the longer-acting insulin last. This is important because longer-acting insulins, if inadvertently added to your vial of regular insulin, can change the activity profile of regular insulins, making them long-acting too. If you were to make this mistake on a regular basis, it could compromise your insulin coverage.

Where Insulin Comes From

Most insulins were once extracted from beef or pork pancreas. These "animal species" insulins differ only slightly from human insulin and act identically to human insulin. Today, however, most doctors prescribe human recombinant insulin to people newly diagnosed with diabetes. Human recombinant insulin is an identical copy of the insulin found in human beings, except that it is produced by bacteria that have been genetically programmed to produce it. It may have a small advantage over beef and pork insulin in that some people with diabetes occasionally have small, localized allergic reactions at the injection sites of animal insulins. Rarely, people with diabetes have serious allergies to beef and pork insulin, and the very strong reactions they have may be life-threatening. The major reason why human insulin was developed was to provide a limitless supply for the world.

People who have used beef or pork insulin successfully over the years should not be switched to human recombinant insulin without good reason. After all, if it ain't broke, don't fix it. Whichever insulin you use, it is generally stable as long as it isn't frozen or boiled. Storing insulin in a refrigerator (not a freezer) is preferred, but it is also quite stable at room temperature.

Insulin Treatment Plans

The ultimate goal of insulin therapy is to provide an insulin level, selected to match your blood sugar level, diet, and exercise, that will maintain your blood sugar in the recommended range. On a daily basis, you should try to avoid wide swings in blood sugar, including hypoglycemia. In the long term, try to keep average blood sugar levels as close to the normal range as possible. There are many, many ways to achieve these goals, and we'll look at them briefly here. Your own insulin treatment plan should be designed individually for you and worked out with all the members of your treatment team. Here are some of the principles of insulin therapy, using the different formulations just described as building blocks.

Insulin Therapy for IDDM

Multiple Daily Injections

Today at Mass General, the most popular insulin treatment plan recommended by doctors is called Multiple Daily Injections, or MDI. The reason it's so popular is because the Diabetes Control and Complications Trial (DCCT) very convincingly showed that, in conjunction with regular consultation with a diabetes treatment team, MDI—or, alternatively, the use of an insulin pump, which we'll discuss later in this chapter—is much more effective in preventing long-term complications than less aggressive insulin treatment plans. You can read all about how much trouble MDI can save you in the long run in Chapter 11, which discusses the DCCT in greater detail.

What the DCCT didn't measure is how much control MDI gives diabetics over their own lives. That's something you'll have to discover by experimenting with different insulin plans under the supervision of your diabetes treatment team.

Multiple Daily Injections sound intimidating, as though you would be injecting yourself ten or twenty times a day. In fact, all it implies is a minimum of three insulin injections combined with frequent attention to monitoring, diet, and exercise (see below). The most common MDI coverage plan requires two or three injections of regular insulin to cover breakfast and dinner, or all three meals, respectively. These doses are adjusted with a "sliding scale" based on your blood glucose levels before the meal. The higher the level and the bigger the meal, the larger the dose. In addition, you may need to take some long- or intermediate-acting insulin in the morning. This can be mixed with your pre-breakfast injection. Finally, you will need an injection of long-acting insulin at dinner or intermediate-acting insulin before bedtime. The long- or inter-

Insulin Treatment Regimens

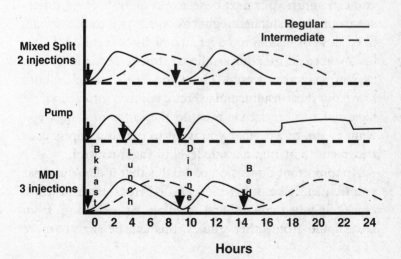

mediate-acting insulin, given once or twice per day, provides the background level of insulin necessary to cover you when your regular insulin is no longer active—especially overnight. You may also need to eat a bedtime snack as a safeguard against hypoglycemia during the night. All these details should be worked out with your treatment team.

It doesn't sound like such a radical plan: injections of rapid-acting insulin for meals, intermediate- or long-acting insulin to provide a basal level of insulin during the day and overnight. Why does it make such a difference in preventing complications? MDI allows you to match your insulin dose to your blood sugar much more closely than older, less natural insulin treatment plans. As you are getting ready for each of your meals, you should be checking your blood sugar, planning your meal, and then taking an appropriate amount of insulin. When you monitor again, before your next meal, or at bedtime, you will have a good idea of how your diet, activity level, and insulin dosage have affected your blood sugar over the last few hours, and you can adjust your next dose accordingly. It's very different from old-fashioned regimens where you took a single, fixed dose of insulin to cover two or three meals. MDI allows you to adjust your insulin treatment frequently, much as your pancreas would. Once you begin to understand how your diet, insulin, and exercise regimen interact, you'll have much more freedom to do the kinds of things you want to do, to eat what you want to eat, and adjust your treatment to maintain a safe level of sugar control.

An important dimension of MDI is that it demands that you frequently consult with your diabetes treatment team, especially when you are first learning. As we've seen from DCCT and from other studies, this can be slightly more expensive than conventional treatment, and the expense may not be covered by all insurance plans. This is unfortunate, because we've shown that MDI can make a big difference in forestalling complications. As we'll see in Chapter 11, we are talking about major reductions in long-term complications and most likely in mortality, as a result of intensive managment.

Education is the key component of any diabetic treatment program. One of my patients was in the Peace Corps when he was diagnosed with type I diabetes at the age of thirty. Now, with his diabetes under control, he wants to

---

Injecting Insulin

People can get very nervous about injecting insulin for the first time. But people can get very nervous about riding a bike or swimming for the first time, too. In all three cases, it's about the same degree of difficulty to get past that first time and go on to becoming proficient.

Mass General sends many children with diabetes to diabetes camp. We have a relationship with Camp Clara Barton, a girl's camp in Oxford, Massachusetts, where I've occasionally spent a day and gotten to know the campers a little bit. I can tell you that it's fun, and very educational. You learn a great deal about how people live with diabetes when you talk to children who have the disease.

On one particular weekend, several grandparents had come to learn more about how to care for children with diabetes. They wanted to be prepared for anything that might come up while they babysat their grandchildren. All these grandparents were interested in spending more time and having more freedom to do things with their grandchildren, and it was great to watch them learn and gain confidence.

(continued)

Injecting Insulin (cont'd)

Most of these grandparents had injected their grandchildren's insulin before, but the camp held a brief refresher course anyway. It was rather simple. We all sat around a table and injected the person on the left, using a small vial of saline and a 0.5-cc syringe.

The best way to learn to inject insulin is on yourself or another person—preferably yourself. Seldom is the procedure taught by sticking a needle into an orange, as it once was, simply because the orange is a poor imitation of the real thing. (I don't know whether the story about the newly instructed diabetic patient who faithfully injected the orange day after day, not understanding why his condition didn't improve, is true or not.) There's very little damage that can be done with an insulin injection, anyway. Here's the procedure, as our teaching nurses usually explain it:

1. Before you do anything, monitor your blood sugar and record it in your diabetes notebook. Then you can start thinking about your injection and the dose you will use.

2. To begin, you need a syringe, a vial of insulin, and an alcohol wipe. Check to make sure it's the right insulin—don't inject NPH when you want to inject regular, or vice versa. Remember to roll the vials of intermediate- or long-acting insulin between your hands.

3. Unwrap the alcohol wipe and clean the top of the insulin vial.

4. Before drawing up the insulin, decide how many units you need. With the syringe uncapped and empty, pull the plunger back to that point, so that you've drawn that number of units of *air* into the barrel.

5. Push the syringe's needle through the rubber cap into the vial, and inject the air into the vial. Now draw up the amount of insulin you've decided upon. The easi-

est way to get the number of units you want accurately is to draw the plunger down *past* the marker
for the number of units you want and then inch it
back slowly up to that point. If you have drawn up
the insulin slowly, there shouldn't be any air bubbles;
however, if there are bubbles, hold the syringe with
the needle pointing up, tap the syringe gently so the
bubbles rise to the top of the barrel, and depress the
plunger to get rid of the air.

6. Pull the needle out of the vial. Now you're ready to
inject the insulin.

7. Grab a fold of skin. If you're injecting insulin into
yourself, an easy place to start is your abdomen or
thigh. If injecting into someone else, a good place is
the back of the upper arm. Don't pinch the skin hard,
just hold it steady. You should have about one inch of
skin visible between your thumb and forefinger. Stay
away from visible blood vessels. Wipe the skin with
your alcohol wipe.

8. Take the syringe between your other thumb and forefinger and push the needle straight into the skin. You
may have seen doctors or nurses put needles in your
arm at an angle. There is no need to do this when you
are injecting *subcutaneously* (under the skin). Push
the syringe down with your thumb. It should prick a
little, but only for a second. Don't be alarmed if a little blood comes out of the injection site. It just means
that you've hit a capillary, a small blood vessel.

9. Wipe the injection site again. Dispose of the needle.
We use an empty coffee can with a small hole cut in
the plastic lid. This makes it harder for small children
to get into the needles and makes disposal easier.

10. Remember to rotate your injection sites based on exercise (see Chapter 6) and avoid using exactly the
same site over and over again.

11. If you are mixing insulin, check with your nurse-
educator to learn the correct technique.

return to Mozambique with the Peace Corps. We had to teach him how to take care of himself in the middle of the jungle with this potentially life-threatening disease. It's difficult, but we did it. More important, you can do it. It just takes some time and effort.

You have to be empowered and taught to care for yourself over a lifetime. This includes everything from emergency care to chronic care. You have to be mindful of the condition of your feet, you have to watch what you eat, you have to control your blood glucose, and you have to monitor. Without you as an active partner, diabetes care, particularly intensive care, will never work.

Insulin Pump

More and more patients are getting interested in insulin pumps for two reasons: pumps are an alternative to injecting insulin, and they can help control blood sugar tightly, facilitating very frequent injections to fine-tune diabetes control.

The insulin pump is a relatively new technology that has come into existence over the past ten to twenty years. The latest pumps are fairly small, about the size of a pager, and just as easy to carry and conceal. They hold a store of rapid-acting insulin that is "pumped" into the body through a small tube attached to a very fine needle, called a catheter. The catheter is inserted into the skin, just like an insulin syringe; however, the catheter is secured in place with a bit of tape and changed every one to two days. Some of my pump-using patients admit to me that they change their catheters only every five days, either because they want to save money or because they get lazy. Leaving the catheter in place for too long can lead to irritation at the needle site and erratic absorption of insulin, or, rarely, a local skin infection.

The interesting thing about the pump is that, more than any other kind of insulin-injection program, it can help you imitate the natural release of insulin that your pancreas would normally provide. This is because the pump is programmed to deliver one long, uninterrupted stream of insulin into your body all day, evening, and night. This is similar to what a normal pancreas does.

Keep in mind that all currently available insulin therapy, including pumps, relies on absorption of insulin from the subcutaneous sites of injection, which leads to a slower appearance and disappearance of insulin than occurs in non-diabetics. In addition, you need to regulate the amount of insulin and the timing of administration in all of the therapies that have been discussed. None of them are automatic.

Before eating meals or snacks, you can program the pump to give you a specific dose of insulin, called a bolus, that will cover the meal. The pump allows you to "bolus" yourself repeatedly during the day without needing to draw up the insulin, find a private place, and inject yourself.

Ralph Dineen has been using the pump for ten years, almost since he was first diagnosed with diabetes. Sometimes, when people who are being treated at Mass General are thinking of going on the pump, they will be referred to Ralph to get a perspective on the pros and cons.

"I'm delighted to talk with anyone who's interested," Ralph says. "I talk to them about pump therapy and what it has meant for me. I'm not trying to sell them on the pump, but just tell them about the effect it has in my life. I have been very pleased to find out that after we talked, some of them have in fact adopted the pump and it seems to be working. That is neat and exciting."

Ralph is a typical pump user in many ways. He is very organized. As an architect, he likes to have a plan and be in control. When I ask Ralph about his pump routine, he is easily able to recite it. As I mentioned above, insulin flows from the pump into the body through a catheter which has to be changed every few days. Ralph sometimes lets it go longer, but that's his own decision. He estimates his monthly costs for catheters and other supplies, including monitoring strips, at around $250. Another expense is the pump itself, which can cost from $2000 to $5000. Insurance often pays for the equipment and supplies.

When Ralph changes his catheter, he usually removes it, showers, and then replaces the catheter when he is done. On days when he doesn't need to change his catheter, Ralph showers with the pump hooked to a chain around his neck. It's important to keep the pump attached to the catheter and functioning *at all times*. For instance, once Ralph was feeling nauseated and couldn't eat anything. Because he couldn't eat, he decided to turn his pump off. That turned out to be a big mistake that led to high blood sugars.

"It was a stupid idea," Ralph says. "Intuitively, it makes sense, because you would normally want to cut down on your insulin if you are not eating anything. The problem is that when you shut the pump down, you begin to deplete the background basal level of insulin that your body needs, whether you are ingesting food or not. The trick is to wait out your nausea, get rid of it, but let your background dose of insulin keep coming into your system. You may even need extra boluses of insulin depending on your blood sugar."

There are some times when Ralph doesn't want to wear his pump, such as when he's at the beach for the summer. For these times, Ralph has found a way to cover his insulin needs while his pump is detached, so that he can go swimming without worrying about the pump.

"I inject myself with a small dose of NPH first thing in the morning and then give myself regular insulin for breakfast and lunch. By the late afternoon, the NPH is wearing off, and I am usually not at the beach anymore. I put the pump back on, give myself a bolus through the pump before dinner, and then go to bed. It works beautifully.

"For me, it was important to figure out the delivery system that would accommodate my level of activity. When I was on summer vacation, I injected insulin during the day and used my pump only in the evening. It worked very well, and it allowed me to keep a routine going. I tried going with multiple injections, four shots a day, and it was more difficult for me to maintain my blood sugars. I found that in the morning my blood sugar was higher than I wanted it to be. To keep my blood sugars down in the early morning, I needed to be on the pump at night. I found out that to make it work, I needed to combine the pump with injections. Then I was able to get the kind of control I wanted, and it was fun to do it. It was like solving a puzzle."

For some people who find it difficult to keep their blood sugar under control, the pump can be a godsend. Wendy Avery Smith, a schoolteacher in a suburb of Boston, started using the pump when she decided she wanted to become pregnant. The pump looked like a way to control her somewhat brittle (especially difficult to control) diabetes.

"Before I started the pump, I might have run a blood sugar of 150 one day, and then over 200 the next. And of course when you're female, there's all this monthly variation, and I'd have to make adjustments, and that was kind of challenging," Wendy recalled. "So after a while, the nurse practitioner mentioned a pump. I still don't have perfect numbers, but they're much better than they used to be."

Wendy became pregnant, kept her blood sugars in near perfect control, and recently gave birth to a healthy baby boy.

Wendy and Ralph and thousands of other persons with type I diabetes have regained control of their day-to-day living by monitoring their diabetes with the use of MDI or insulin pumps. *They* control their diabetes, not vice versa. Although the methods they use are far better than those available twenty years ago, the intensive treatments still require a substantial commitment of energy, if not time.

A number of companies are currently experimenting with implantable pumps that are surgically placed beneath the surface of the skin and can be programmed with a small transmitter. The advantage to this system is that it is totally implanted and eliminates the need to carry an external pump, or to inject. The drawback to these experimental pumps is that they are still somewhat large, about the size of a hockey puck. Laura Barrus is a nurse at Mass General whose pump was implanted a little over two years ago. She was very excited about her implantable pump, and really enjoyed the freedom and convenience of not having to inject insulin or change catheters. The real breakthrough with these devices will come when automatic glucose monitoring is developed and connected to the pumps. Then, they will be capable of providing the right dose of insulin automatically. These true artificial pancreata will make diabetes care safe, foolproof, and more user-friendly than the currently available methods.

Split-Mixed Programs

As I have said, MDI is more or less the gold standard for insulin treatment plans for type I diabetes. It's currently advocated by doctors at Mass General because it has been shown that an aggressive approach to treating diabetes can lead to a much lower risk of complications.

Still, there are many people with IDDM who find it difficult or impossible to commit themselves to three or more daily injections of insulin or to an insulin pump. Alternatively, there may be some people with IDDM whose risk for hypoglycemia is so great, or whose level of complications is sufficiently advanced, that intensive therapy doesn't make sense. For these people, a more simple, less demanding insulin plan is appropriate. One of the ways to reduce the number of injections is to give two daily injections of mixed insulins, usually NPH and regular (see the figure on p. 99). In this manner, the number of injections can be cut to two. The doses of insulin can still be adjusted based on monitoring results and other factors.

Typically, one injection of regular insulin and NPH is given at breakfast, and another at dinnertime. The regular insulin you take in your first injection will cover your breakfast, while the NPH from that same injection will peak in the middle of the afternoon, covering your lunch. The second injection of regular insulin will cover your dinner, while the NPH should help control blood sugar levels throughout the night, although usually not as effectively as bedtime NPH in an MDI program.

At first, it may seem that taking two daily injections gives you much more freedom than three or four. However, the drawback to such programs is that although they look easier, they are actually less flexible, often obligating you to eat extra snacks to prevent hypoglycemia. In addition, two-injection regimens usually can't achieve the lower level of blood sugar control necessary to prevent long-term complications.

Single Injection

Most patients with IDDM who take single injections of insulin and maintain acceptable blood sugar levels have some measure of pancreatic function remaining and just need to supplement the amount of insulin they are able to generate on their own. This category includes some people newly diagnosed with IDDM. After newly diagnosed people with IDDM begin taking insulin, they often go through a period when their insulin output rises (or their insulin requirements fall) to a level where they almost don't need injections anymore. This diabetes "honeymoon" period can last up to a year, sometimes even longer. As long as the honeymoon period lasts, a person with IDDM may need to fill only a percentage of his or her needs by insulin injection, letting the pancreas itself do the fine adjusting.

People with NIDDM, as we will discuss later, often take only one daily injection of insulin, because their pancreata are still working, albeit insufficiently. Their insulin needs may be very great, however, because they may suffer from something called insulin resistance. This means that their bodies do not respond to insulin as readily as they once did, and they need more insulin to get the same blood-sugar-lowering effect.

Insulin for NIDDM

Although not insulin-dependent by definition, the majority of patients using insulin have NIDDM, not IDDM. This reflects the common occurrence of NIDDM compared with the relatively rare occurrence of IDDM (about 8 million diagnosed with NIDDM versus less than 1 million IDDM patients in the United States) and the eventual failure of diet and oral agents to control glucose adequately in NIDDM. The reason to aim for normal glucose control in NIDDM is the same as in IDDM—the hope that long-term complications will be prevented or reduced. In any case, many NIDDM patients are eventually treated with insulin (the treatments specific to NIDDM are addressed in Chapter 10). While the types of insulin used in the therapy of NIDDM are the same as for IDDM, the way in which they are used is different.

Because people with NIDDM continue to make some of their own insulin, blood sugar levels are usually more stable than they are in people with IDDM. Thus, people with NIDDM are able to use simpler insulin replacement schedules than those with IDDM. Controlling blood sugars in the near-normal range requires multiple daily injections in IDDM; however, in NIDDM, only one or two daily injections are usually all that is necessary. The insulin, usually intermediate-acting or mixed intermediate- and rapid-acting, can be given in the morning. Alternatively, intermediate-acting insulin can be given at bedtime. Many insulin regimens have been used successfully in NIDDM.

IDDM or NIDDM: Am I Insulin-Dependent?

In all of diabetes terminology, perhaps nothing is as confusing as the distinction between insulin-dependent diabetes mellitus (IDDM or type I) and non-insulin-dependent diabetes mellitus (NIDDM or type II). The distinction is not simply, "one takes insulin, the other doesn't."

The key is in the concept of dependency. People with IDDM have lost the function of their beta cells, the cells in the pancreas that produce insulin. They are totally dependent on injected insulin because they don't make any of their own. Without the injected insulin, they develop ketoacidosis in one to two days, and they can die if not treated.

People with NIDDM can make their own insulin and often make a lot of it. Their problem lies in their increased need for insulin, which they cannot match. It is a problem of supply and demand—they need more than they can make. Therefore, many people with NIDDM need extra insulin to control their blood sugar levels, but they are not usually at risk for ketoacidosis if they miss their insulin dosage, because they still make some insulin on their own.

As described in Chapter 1, these two forms of diabetes have different causes and people with them usually "look" different. IDDM is an autoimmune disease where the body's immune system destroys the insulin-producing cells of the pancreas. People with IDDM are usually young when they get it. The cause of NIDDM is more mysterious, but it is not autoimmune. People with NIDDM are usually older and heavier at the time of diagnosis than people with IDDM.

The key to achieving acceptable blood glucose control in NIDDM is to use *enough* insulin. The total daily dose that is required often exceeds 50 units, and can run into the hundreds of units. If you think of the insulin dose as being proportional to your body weight, the larger doses of insulin needed to treat NIDDM are not unexpected—bigger people, more insulin.

Interestingly, severe hypoglycemia (low blood sugar) seems to be much less common in insulin-treated persons with NIDDM compared with insulin therapy in persons with IDDM. Hopefully, this should reassure both patients and health care professionals that they can use the large doses required to achieve acceptable glucose control. Monitoring glucose levels for safety and to guide the choice of insulin doses is recommended; however, insulin doses in NIDDM tend to be more stable than in IDDM. The doses often remain stable for long periods of time. Attention to diet remains critical when NIDDM patients are treated with insulin. Some patients think that they can ignore their diet when insulin is started because they are now on a "powerful" medicine and diets are no longer necessary. Unfortunately, this is not the case. As insulin is adjusted, patients will often gain a modest amount of weight. This occurs because the calories they were previously wasting in the form of sugar in the urine are no longer being excreted. This weight gain can be limited or even eliminated if dietary restriction is continued.

6

Exercise: Discover Your Own Fitness Prescription

Exercise has been recognized as the third "leg" of diabetes care for more than seventy years, yet it's often the last thing we think of when designing a treatment plan. It's interesting that whenever we talk about the classical self-treatment triangle (monitoring should now be added as a fourth leg), exercise always brings up the rear. Your diabetologist, diabetes educator, and dietitian may talk to you about exercise, but all too commonly, it's the last thing they bring up, too. Why does exercise get left off the agenda so often?

First of all, many diabetics feel uncomfortable with the idea of exercise, and may even fear working out. A recent national study showed that diabetics were significantly less likely to say that they had recently exercised than people without the disease. Also, people with diabetes were much more likely to report walking as exercise than people without diabetes, who reported more strenuous forms of exercise, such as jogging, swimming, and bicycling.

People with diabetes need to know more about exercise before they feel comfortable engaging in it. You know that physical activity can cause your blood sugar to drop, but how much and for how long? No one enjoys insulin reactions, especially in public, and so a lot of people who take insulin would rather just avoid exercise than take the chance of finding themselves out on a basketball court with a low blood sugar.

Another reason has to do with traditional approaches to diabetic treatment. There are many specialists who can counsel us in our use of monitoring, food, and medications. But there is seldom anyone on the treatment team who specializes in providing exercise programs to persons with diabetes. Although most care providers would like their patients with diabetes to exercise, they don't have formal training in the area, and they tend to shy away from giving any specific guidance about it. Also, complications that commonly accompany diabetes—kidney problems, eye disease, and abnormalities in nerve function—require modifications of the exercise prescription. Finally, more advanced complications of diabetes, such as amputations, loss of vision, and heart disease, interfere with the ability to do certain types of exercise.

Another possible reason is that exercise isn't absolutely necessary. What I mean is that in order to live, you must eat, and in order to live as a person with IDDM, you must manage your insulin. But you can probably get away without an exercise program. Most care providers look at exercise as something that has to be *accounted for* with diet and insulin, rather than as a consistently used *component* of the diabetic treatment program.

But for people with IDDM, skipping exercise means missing out on something with great potential to make life more enjoyable. Fear of low blood sugars or other problems arising from exercise can keep you from indulging in this important part of life—or you can overcome those fears and start reaping the *benefits* of exercise as part of your self-treatment plan.

If you have NIDDM, the chances are high that you are also overweight. Most emphasis has been placed on dietary approaches to help you lose. However, recent research has identified exercise as an important component of weight-loss programs. At the very least, exercise may help you get past the "plateau" of weight loss. This common phenomenon occurs after several weeks to months on a previously effective diet, when people often notice that their weight loss stops, even though they're maintaining the same low caloric intake. This is because your body readjusts its metabolism after the initial weight loss so that it burns off fewer calories. Since reducing dietary calories even further is often difficult, exercise can be used to increase the calories you burn off and restart your weight loss.

In any case, exercise is generally effective in helping you lose and maintain your weight. I'm also convinced that people who successfully build exercise into their daily schedules find it easier to organize their entire treatment programs. Finally, and perhaps most important, exercise improves both peripheral circulation (in your legs) and cardiac conditioning.

Since people with NIDDM, being generally older than those with IDDM, are more likely to have underlying heart disease, they must consult their health care provider before changing their exercise level. Remember that increasing activity level doesn't mean you have to take up beach volleyball or power lifting; a twenty-minute walk each evening might do the trick.

If you're not already used to exercising, it may be hard to get into the habit. Some of the things that people find most unpleasant about exercise are pain, fatigue, and a sense that they're wasting time. So, my advice to people who don't have much experience with exercise is to try to make it a small but consistent part of their daily lives. For example, suppose you work on the fifth floor of a building, and you frequently have to speak with people who work on the seventh floor. Start by walking those stairs, rather than taking the elevator. You'll be amazed at how much time you'll save by not waiting for the elevator anymore and you probably won't miss the glares of the elevator riders who have been stopping at *every* floor to let out passengers who wouldn't walk one or two flights.

Generally speaking, there's no better way to start exercising than walking. It's easy, it doesn't require any special equipment, the risk of injury is minimal, and if you get tired you can always sit down and catch your breath. And your body responds to exercise very promptly: it may be difficult to walk up two flights of stairs on Monday, but if you do it every day of the week, it will be a breeze by Friday. In general, most experts think that you need to walk or exercise briskly enough to break a sweat to get the benefits of exercise. Several studies have shown that performing this level of exercise three to four times per week reduces the risk of heart disease. Of course, any increase in calorie expenditure will help with weight control. The real challenge is to do it regularly and not find excuses— bad weather, needing new sneakers, not wanting to miss favorite TV shows—to avoid exercise.

Before Exercising

When children enter a school athletic program, the school usually demands that they undergo a medical examination. In fact, anyone who wants to start exercising regularly should check with his or her doctor first. This is particularly important for people with diabetes. If you have IDDM, you may need an adjustment in insulin. If you have NIDDM, you may need to adjust your medications, and your doctor will need to make sure you don't have any type of heart disease that may impose restrictions. With either form of diabetes, foot care and appropriate footwear are particularly important, especially if you have neuropathy (abnormal nerve function).

Talk to your doctor before starting your exercise program. Evaluate your current self-treatment program, and talk about your goals for blood sugar control. While you're at it, have your heart function and eyes checked, just to get a status report.

If you use insulin, you should check your blood sugar before engaging in any strenuous exercise, such as running, playing tennis, or swimming. If your blood sugar is normal, you should keep something sweet handy, in case you need to eat. If your sugar is low, eat something and wait until your blood sugar climbs—twenty to thirty minutes should do it— before exercising. Remember that low blood glucose levels may occur during exercise, but they often crop up hours after your exertions are over. Check your blood sugar carefully any time you've exerted yourself in an unaccustomed manner.

You should avoid strenuous exercise if your glucose levels are particularly high, and especially if you are dehydrated or have ketones in your urine. If your monitor reads over 250, check immediately for ketones in your urine. Avoid strenuous exercise under these conditions, since exercise may worsen, not improve, your blood sugar. Get your blood sugar under control, and consult your treatment team before going further with your exercise program.

Remember: exercise is tough on your feet. Make sure you're wearing comfortable shoes that fit, and check your feet after you've finished exercising. Never break in new shoes with exercise. Also, if you're going to be exercising alone, running in the park, for example, you should always wear a Medicalert bracelet in case of emergency. Finally, if you have severe retinopathy (eye disease), some forms of high-impact exercise, like diving or football, may cause bleeding in the back of your eye. It's best to consult your health care professional or ophthalmologist (if you have had laser treatment) before beginning these potentially injurious forms of exercise.

If you incorporate exercise into your daily routine, it seems less like work. Once you've started to think about that walk upstairs as part of your routine, you've made an important shift in your thinking. You may be ready to take an evening constitutional at a brisk pace, or to take up aerobics, dancing, or swimming. You'll see that your new exercise regimen improves your mood, your stamina, and your feelings about your body and even about yourself.

If you take insulin or sulfonylureas, you may need to adjust your doses. Although a modest decrease in insulin is often appropriate, the type of insulin that needs to be adjusted and the amount of the dosage is different for everyone. A patient at Mass General provided me with an excellent example of how to cope with this problem. Ralph Dineen, whom we met in the previous chapter, is on an insulin pump, so he's receiving a constant, low "basal rate" of insulin all day long (see Chapter 5). Before meals, he uses the Carbo Counting System (see Chapter 4) to calculate how much coverage he needs and gives himself a "bolus" of insulin with the pump.

On Saturdays, Ralph likes to eat and enjoy himself. So his wife mixes up a big batch of french toast with real maple syrup. Normally, Ralph takes his bolus of insulin half an hour before a meal, and on Saturdays, he raises the bolus by three units. He sits down with his wife and children and eats his french toast with real maple syrup and then goes out and rakes some leaves and works in the yard all day long. Although Ralph *thinks* that everything is going to be okay—because he has experimented with this and he knows that three units will cover him—he still checks his glucose levels more frequently on these days to make sure that they remain in a safe, acceptable range.

You don't need an insulin pump to achieve this kind of control. You just need to look at exercise as part of your daily life and understand that it's going to have an effect on your blood sugar. Once you understand what that effect is, exercise becomes much less complicated. If you can plan and anticipate your exercise, making the necessary adjustments is easier.

Meryl Cohen has been a physical therapist for twenty years and has always worked with patients in need of acute care. For most of that time, she has focused on working with people suffering from heart disease, and a number of these people have also had diabetes. Meryl had always wanted to be part of an organized effort to get people with diabetes into exercise programs, so she arranged a program at Mass General.

"We try to show patients how much their blood glucose level drops with exercise," she says. "We try to develop individualized plans, but we can also help people exercise in groups. Our main goal is to get our people to exercise daily for an hour. It's important to exercise regularly, because exercise changes insulin requirements. If you stop exercising and fail to make up for it with insulin, it could cause your blood sugar to jump."

For many of the same reasons that we listed above, Cohen has found that most of her patients need to be educated about exercise at a very basic level. Many of them are uncomfortable with the idea of exercise to start with. However, they all want to take care of their diabetes, and they are willing to try new things and expend a little effort if they think it will help them feel more healthy, self-confident, and in control of their diabetes.

"The first week I spend with someone, I like to get to know them a little bit and learn about their capacity for exercise," Meryl says. She likes to start people off with easy walking exercises or riding a stationary bicycle. These are things that almost anyone can do for at least a few minutes. Because most of the people she works with have other medical problems, Cohen monitors their heart rate and blood pressure.

You can monitor your own heart rate by taking your pulse. Simply place the tips of your first and second fingers on your opposite wrist, just below the thumb. You can usually find the pulse by feeling around for a second or two. Another good pulse spot is in your neck, right below the angle of your jawbone. Press your index and middle fingers lightly on either of those spots, and count beats while you time for fifteen seconds. Then multiply by four.

A healthy, resting heart rate can be anywhere from 50 to 100 beats per minute, depending on the individual. You can monitor your pulse to make sure that you're not overdoing—or underdoing—your exercise. If you're concerned about overdoing it, there are some simple formulas for making sure that your heart is working at a safe but healthy pace. This is called finding your target heart rate.

Target Heart Rate

The target heart rate is a useful tool to make sure that the intensity of your exercise is reasonably consistent. To calculate your target heart rate, begin by subtracting your age from 220. I'm forty-six, so 220−46=174. Now, if you're just beginning an exercise program, you should take about 55 to 60 percent of that number as your target heart rate. When I'm starting an exercise program, my target heart rate would be a little more than half of 174, or about 100. So until I felt a little more comfortable exercising, I would try to do a workout that would raise my pulse to about 100 beats per minute.

A good rule of thumb is to always make sure that you can talk comfortably when exercising. If you're panting too much to speak, you're working too hard.

As your stamina increases, you may be able to increase your target heart rate for workouts, to 70 and then maybe 80 percent of the original number that you got when you subtracted your age from 220. It's probably unwise to go much past 90 percent of that original number.

If you have any history of or worries about vision problems, heart disease, neuropathy, or kidney disease, DO NOT begin exercising without consulting your diabetologist. In any case, it's always a good idea to consult with your treatment team before starting an exercise program, because they can help you make modifications in your diet and medication program that will help you avoid hypoglycemia. And they'll probably give you all kinds of encouragement, too.

The target heart rate is not a hard-and-fast rule but a target you set for yourself when you're exercising. If you keep to a fairly consistent heart rate, you'll be better able to regulate how hard you exercise.

One of the hardest parts of exercising is getting people to take the first step. So Meryl Cohen has several approaches to exercise that appeal to different people. In general, she encourages them to begin exercise with meth-

---

Pre-Exercise Injection Sites

Before you start to work out, think about the muscles that will be doing the most work. If you'll be doing sit-ups, it will be your abdomen; if walking, your legs and buttocks; if tennis, your dominant arm.

Insulin is absorbed faster through muscles that are working hard. The muscle activity will carry your insulin dose into your system faster, and your insulin will peak more quickly than usual, sometimes much more quickly.

Choose an injection site where muscles probably won't be working so hard. If you're going for a walk, inject your insulin into your arm or abdomen; tennis players should inject either the abdomen or the arm that doesn't swing the tennis racket. This will allow your insulin to reach your bloodstream on its regular timetable.

---

ods that are readily available, user-friendly, and fun. Walking with a friend is always easy, and your exercise tolerance may improve even more if you talk the whole time you're walking. If you have access to a tennis court, treadmill, or bike, you can find ways to work a quick game, jog, or ride into your schedule.

Meryl also recommends that some of her patients exercise with a Theraband—an elastic band that can be stretched between the hands or between hands and feet. The set of bands are color coded for their varying resistances, so that you can work your way up to a harder workout through the different bands. They're small, very portable, and not at all conspicuous, so they can go in a suitcase on a business trip for use in a hotel room.

It's that kind of adaptability and ease of use that Meryl looks for in exercise equipment. "People will look for any excuse not to exercise," she says with a knowing smile. "You've got to make it as simple as possible."

Another tool she likes to use is the portable step. You can keep a portable step under the bed, or in a closet, and it's very easy to slide out and set up. Using a step, you can very quickly raise your heart rate to a desired level and keep it there, and there's little risk of hurting yourself or falling. Of course, you can go up and down a staircase, but stepping is an easy exercise that you can do while following an aerobics video or watching a movie on TV—whatever motivates you.

"A lot of people need a buddy to exercise with," adds Cohen. "Find a buddy and walk at a mall, a health club, anywhere the weather can't interfere with your schedule." Your buddy could be a friend, a coworker, a spouse—not necessarily someone with diabetes—preferably someone whose schedule is compatible with yours so that you can have a regular routine, and someone who will share with you the responsibility of reminding and motivating.

You really ought to take it easy as you are becoming accustomed to exercise. But once you get going, there's really little limit to what you can do, provided your doctor gives you the go-ahead. People with diabetes play competitive sports and engage in strenuous exercise at all levels. The Phoenix-based International Diabetes Athletic Association (IDAA) supports and encourages people with diabetes who want to make the most of their physical lives. The group runs conferences and workshops at which people with diabetes can learn about how to manage their diabetes while exercising. These are some common questions:

- How can I work out with food in my stomach?
- Do I have to work out at the same time and with the same intensity each day?

Paula Harper, R.N., C.D.E., president of the IDAA, founded the group in 1985 hoping that with education and research, more people with diabetes would gain access to exercise programs, make exercise part of their regular routines, and reap health benefits. Here is her account of how she started out almost twenty years ago.

I embarked on a running program in 1976 with little information about how it would affect my type I diabetes (IDDM). I developed a training regimen to build my endurance, and within one year, I entered my first marathon race. I went on to complete thirty more marathons, one ultramarathon (50 miles), as well as five triathlons, and six century (100-plus miles) bicycle races. That was quite an athletic feat for someone who previously was not big on exercise. The problem came when I sought medical advice for training. I was most often given inadequate or misleading advice. . . . I was troubled to learn that doctors had little helpful advice and were generally unwilling to work with me.

I set out on training runs, kept good records to chart my progress, and learned the most by trial and error. In retrospect, what I did seems scary. These were the days before home blood glucose monitoring, and I am sure that there were times when I exercised with my blood glucose too high or too low. With miles to go in one marathon, I had exhausted my supply of sugar-containing snacks and was experiencing low blood glucose because of poor advice [from] my physician about the amount of insulin to take for this endurance event. I was urged to drop out of the race. I would not think of it. Someone at an aid station gave me a soda, a policeman gave me a pack of chewing gum, and I crossed the finish line feeling better than I had during the middle of the race. Granted, this is not the optimal plan for running a twenty-six-mile distance, but it worked. I was not fast, but I was never a quitter.

"I Run on Insulin" became my byword. I had it printed

on the back of a race shirt, and, to my surprise, when I wore it in races, I made many new friends who also had diabetes and endured similar problems. This growing network of active people with diabetes was actually the first step in starting the IDAA. I learned of many young athletes who were being kept from participation because of coaches' fears of difficulties with blood glucose regulation, and I realized the need for education and the crime in turning off youngsters to sports. I feel that the characteristics that allow an athlete to compete successfully and also to maintain good blood glucose control are essentially identical:

1. The desire to do the job right (the ability to make a short- and long-term commitment to learn about the disease continually and to make the adjustments in lifestyle that are required for excellent glucose control).
2. An understanding of how the game is played and what must be done to succeed (detailed knowledge of the pathophysiology of diabetes, the various types of insulin and their actions, and the effects of diet and exercise on blood glucose regulation).
3. The discipline to do what is needed consistently to succeed (to monitor blood glucose methodically multiple times daily, to avoid unhealthy diet and activity patterns, while making healthy alternatives a routine part of one's daily life).
4. Skill (the ability to check blood glucose accurately and to choose the appropriate dietary manipulations to prevent major swings in blood glucose before, during, and after exercise).

There are chapters of the IDAA across the United States, in Europe, Canada, and Japan.

A member of the Swedish national soccer team that came to the 1994 World Cup competition in the United States has IDDM. This twenty-four-year-old is competing at an international level in what could be considered the world's most demanding competitive professional sport. It's estimated that soccer players run an average of eight miles during ninety minutes of nonstop competition, with only a brief rest during halftime. If diabetes were going to stand in the way of a sport, this would probably be the one. But that's not the nature of diabetes. The disease doesn't get in the way of exercise as much as its complications do, and your best bet at preventing complications is to control your blood sugar *and* get plenty of exercise.

There is no reason for you to think that simply having diabetes eliminates your athletic potential, no matter what your age, weight, height, or sex. Many of my patients with diabetes scuba dive, wrestle, bike, run marathons and even participate in grueling triathlons. One of our patients, Dr. David Henderson, a retired geographer who lives in New Bedford, Massachusetts, said that in his early twenties he spent days and weeks on horseback during geographical expeditions in Mexico. He monitored his blood sugar daily—albeit with now-outdated urine-testing methods—and was always able to control insulin reactions with the fruits or sweets he carried with him.

Dr. Henderson says that one of his closest friends, a classmate from his youth, also has IDDM. He continues to ski in his seventies, and he also carries fruit with him at all times to treat low blood sugars. Both these people with diabetes have made exercise an integral part of their lives, something that they have not allowed diabetes to take away from them.

You don't have to run marathons or play World Cup soccer for your diabetes control to benefit from exercise. Any regular program that gets your pulse in its target range for twenty to thirty minutes, three or four times a week, will work for you. Even brisk walking can do this. But if a tough, competitive sport is what you crave, it's nice to know that many other people with diabetes have successfully taken that road. If you follow several important do's and don'ts, your exercise will be safe, beneficial, and pleasurable.

Do's and Don'ts of Exercise in Diabetes

- Do include exercise as part of your daily life.
- Do plan exercise as much as possible so that you can adjust your therapy.
- Do consider changes in insulin dose, injection site, and snacking to adjust for exercise and prevent hypoglycemia.
- Do discuss changes in exercise patterns with your physician.
- Do pay particular attention to foot care with exercise.
- Don't exercise if your blood sugar is in poor control.
- Don't exercise before consulting your physician, especially if you have a history or symptoms of heart disease, eye disease, or abnormal nerve function.

7

Hypoglycemia

"It's the middle of the night, the room is pitch black, and I wake up realizing that something is not quite right. The baby is lying in a crib next to the bed, stirring slightly, and Judi seems not to have responded. She must be tired, I tell myself, and try to wake her.

"Judi rolls over in bed, opens her eyes, and says, 'Okay, okay, I'm up.' Assuming that she's about to start feeding the baby, I put my head down and think about going back to sleep. But the crying goes on and Judi doesn't move—she continues to stare at the ceiling. I start to sense that something is wrong.

" 'Are you low?' I ask, and I wipe my hand across her abdomen to see whether she's sweaty. Her skin is slightly damp, but it could just be the warmth of the covers. 'I'm okay, I'm okay,' she says. But it doesn't sound like Judi to me, her voice sounds wooden and distant.

" 'Well, I think you're low,' I say, and as I get up, I decide to start treating Judi for a low blood sugar reaction. In the meantime, James has begun screaming in earnest. I pick him out of the crib and walk to the kitchen where I run a cold glass of water mixed with two tablespoonfuls of sugar. I've already made up my mind that Judi is very low, and I don't have any glucagon because she had another hypoglycemic episode only a few days before and we used up our last kit. I don't want to take any chances of her losing consciousness, because if that happens, the next step is to call an ambulance. I don't want to spend the rest of the night in the emergency room, and I really don't want for Judi to be sick.

"As I give Judi her first drink of sugar water, it's 2:28 A.M. I know that if she hasn't responded by 2:48 at the latest, I'll have to give her more sugar. She sits up in bed, and I give her the sugar water to sip.

"In the meantime, the baby's cries have become one long loud scream. I know that Judi's still hypoglycemic, because of her indifference toward James. Her attitude is that of a child seeing a frog for the first time: the mildest of interest, and a hint of distaste. But this doesn't last long. Within five minutes of drinking the sugar water, Judi says simply: 'Give him to me.' And I know that she's back."

This is the story of low blood sugar, or hypoglycemia, from someone who has watched his spouse go through the experience. I can only imagine how frightening it must be for the people who face this possibility every day of their lives. Several times, people with diabetes have remarked to me, "I lost an hour there": they were unable to remember anything that happened while hypoglycemic. Their first recollections are of friends, loved ones, or strangers standing by them, anxiously awaiting their return from this distant, frightening state. Even more disturbing are the episodes in which patients find themselves parked in their driveways, unable to recall driving home from work.

Other people with diabetes have talked about the embarrassment, the fear of hypoglycemia. They have experienced the frustration of trying to make people understand that they need something to eat, right away, that they're not drunk or psychotic, they just need something sweet and they'll be fine, and that they don't mean to be cranky or short tempered.

However humiliating it may be to suffer a hypoglycemic episode in front of friends, or even total strangers, there is an even greater potential for serious problems. I've talked to patients who have had low blood sugars behind the wheel: sometimes they can't remember pulling over to the side of the road. I've heard from patients who've awakened alone in their beds, unable to move or speak. People have told me stories of crawling to the refrigerator, struggling to swallow a mouthful of juice. Some have fallen down and been injured, or worse.

What is hypoglycemia? Although the specific manifestations of a hypoglycemic episode may differ from person to person, may change over time, and may not occur at the same level of blood sugar for all people, in general, hypoglycemia occurs when the brain is not supplied with enough of its main fuel, glucose. Although once a fad condition among people *without* diabetes, hypoglycemia is a continuing reality for anyone *with* diabetes who is treated with insulin or sulfonylureas.

Blood sugar levels below the body's normal range can bring on several symptoms that presage more serious effects. The first sign of low blood glucose is usually the development of symptoms, such as a rapid heartbeat with palpitations, sweating, tremulousness, and the feeling that something isn't right. These symptoms are caused by the release of *adrenaline,* a hormone that people produce when they perceive that they are threatened or in danger, or are stressed.

Feeling like this tells you that your sugar level is dropping and that you should eat something sweet, right away. You have to add sugar quickly to your bloodstream to prevent your blood sugar from dipping even lower. The relatively mild, albeit uncomfortable, symptoms associated with the early stages of hypoglycemia can become more severe if you don't get treatment rapidly enough, or if you don't raise your blood sugar level enough to restore normal function. The later, more severe stages of hypoglycemia include altered mental function with confusion, double vision, slurred speech, and poor balance. They're similar to the effects of drinking alcohol to excess. If your blood sugar falls low enough, you may experience loss of consciousness or seizures.

Unfortunately, there is no exact number on your glucose monitor that announces: "You're hypoglycemic." The low end of the normal range of blood sugar for most people lies somewhere between 55 and 65 mg/dl. However, there are many people who continue to function normally well below that range, and who probably don't feel symptomatic until going below 60 mg/dl, or even much lower. On the other hand, people with diabetes whose blood sugars tend to run high chronically say that they may start feeling sweaty or confused when their blood sugar drops below 75 mg/dl.

To add to the confusion, the level of blood glucose that causes clinical symptoms of hypoglycemia early on in the course of insulin-dependent diabetes (IDDM) may not cause warning symptoms after you have had diabetes for five or ten years. Moreover, the symptoms that occur with hypoglycemia change and become more subtle over time. After five to ten years of diabetes, people often note that reactions tend to sneak up on them, leaving them little time to treat themselves before confusion, or, even worse, unconsciousness, makes it difficult or impossible for them to respond appropriately. Finally, the intensive therapy that so effectively reduces risk for long-term complications of diabetes lowers the threshold of the level of blood sugar at which you experience warning symptoms. For example, instead of experiencing warning symptoms at a blood sugar of 60 mg/dl—which would be more likely to happen if your blood sugars were in poorer control—keeping your sugars under tight control might mean that you would feel no symptoms at all until your blood sugar had reached 30 or 40 mg/dl. This gives you less time to respond. The cause for these changes isn't entirely clear but we now know that episodes of low blood sugar tend to lead to the changes above. In other words, hypoglycemic episodes beget more hypoglycemic episodes.

Many people with diabetes would rather suffer the consequences of chronic high blood sugar levels than have an insulin reaction; they prove it by running their sugars high all the time, thus making hypoglycemia a more remote possibility. Of course, we now know that anyone who does this increases the risk of developing complications, such as eye and kidney disease.

How do you strike a happy medium? Is it possible to keep blood sugars at a safe, healthy level while avoiding hypoglycemia? I don't know for sure. The Diabetes Control and Complications Trial kept track of hypoglycemic episodes in both treatment groups, one of which was attempting to control blood sugar tightly, and the other of which was not. The group in tight control experienced three times as many insulin reactions as the group that was not attempting to keep tight control. However, most of the people who had these reactions responded quickly to treatment at home or work, and they rarely suffered loss of consciousness or seizures (an average of one episode every six to seven years of intensive therapy). There were no deaths, heart attacks, or strokes that could be attributable to hypoglycemia.

If you have trouble with insulin reactions, there are a few things you can look for in your routine that may have caused them. In particular, look for reasons that the amount of insulin you took didn't match your insulin needs. Ask yourself if one of these things happened over the past few hours:

• Did you skip a meal, or eat more lightly than usual? If you came up short of your usual calorie count, but took the same amount of insulin, you will probably have a blood sugar that is at least somewhat lower than usual (see Chapter 4).

• Did you take more insulin than usual? Or did you take a greater dose of oral medication than you usually take? If you took more insulin than usual, but the same amount of food, that could also lower your blood sugar (see Chapter 5).

• Did you exercise or exert yourself more than usual? Exercise takes sugar out of your bloodstream; it can also cause your insulin to peak faster than usual, which will contribute to lowering your blood sugar (see Chapter 6).

Detecting hypoglycemia in children can be difficult, particularly when you've never seen it before. Children react to low blood sugar in many different ways, some by acting sleepy, others with violence. A child who is confused may vigorously resist eating anything. Carmella

Clark told me that her baby, Jessie, would most often react to a low blood sugar by crying. She checks Jessie's sugar every night before going to bed.

"This poor kid is tired and sometimes when she is low she has to eat ice cream," Carmella says. "I have to say 'No, Jessie, you cannot go to bed, you have to eat.'

"I remember once we had to get her up and feed her orange juice at 2:30 in the morning because she was low. As a parent, you think that this is not a normal thing, but you still have to deal with it and do it. But she was happy to be eating because obviously she could feel that there was a problem, too."

If your child has diabetes, be sure to keep anyone who regularly supervises him or her, especially babysitters and teachers, well informed. Let them know at what time of day your child is at the greatest risk for getting low and the best way to recognize it, whether it's sleepiness, belligerence, or silliness. Make sure they have telephone numbers so they can call you or your child's doctor in case of emergency. Tell them how you treat low blood sugars at home, and, if possible, give them the kind of sugar source you use to treat hypoglycemia.

Symptoms of Hypoglycemia

People who have been recently diagnosed often have a great fear of low blood sugars. It's only natural: no one likes to lose self-control, let alone lose consciousness. You can usually spot the onset of hypoglycemia if you can identify one or a combination of these symptoms:

- sweating
- shaking
- hunger

- rapid and/or irregular heartbeat
- headache

Some people have their own tip-offs for recognizing hypoglycemia. As the early-warning symptoms of hypoglycemia wane with advanced diabetes, several of my patients have told me that they have a feeling of numbness around the mouth, or double vision, when they're hypoglycemic. Other people have told me that they know they're getting low when they suddenly can't remember a word or the name of a familiar street. Keep in mind that as time goes on, symptoms of hypoglycemia may become more subtle, and you'll have to be more attentive to them. Frequent monitoring will become much more important as a way of protecting yourself from low blood sugars. It is also important to educate the people around you so that they can help you identify the symptoms. If a low blood sugar level goes untreated, then more severe symptoms may begin to occur, and the person with hypoglycemia may be unable to treat him- or herself. The symptoms that reflect decreased glucose delivery to the brain include the following:

- personality changes, including confusion, belligerence, obstinacy
- indifference to crisis
- slurred speech
- double vision
- unconsciousness
- seizure

Treating Hypoglycemia

The best treatment for hypoglycemia is—surprise!—sugar. "Ah-ha," you're saying, "this is the kind of treatment

I can live with. Finally, a disease where the cure tastes great."

When any one of the warning flags is raised, you don't need your monitor. Quickly take a snack that offers readily available carbohydrate: four to six ounces of fruit juice, soda *(not diet soda),* some candy—anything with some sugar in it. Ralph Dineen, the architect we met in Chapter 5, told me that he found skim milk can ward off mild hypoglycemia. The reduced fat allows you to absorb the sugar in the milk more quickly.

Indeed, there is nothing quite like sugar for hypoglycemia. I always advise people to keep hard candy, sugar cubes, a tube of cake icing, a small container of juice, or anything sweet and portable with them so that they can treat themselves immediately if they feel the early symptoms of low blood sugar coming on.

However, don't fall into the trap of thinking that hypoglycemia is your ticket to food paradise. As appealing as it may be to use the treatment of hypoglycemia as an excuse to eat the sweets that you usually limit or deny yourself, a hypoglycemic episode should be treated as a medical condition. The sugar or soda you take to abort the episode is your medicine.

There are a few simple rules for treating hypoglycemia that you ought to drill into yourself, mainly because there may be times when you're so confused by hypoglycemia that you're not sure what you're doing. Many people have told me about suddenly finding themselves at the refrigerator, drinking a glass of juice, unable to remember how they got there. They had treated so many previous hypoglycemic episodes in the same way that they acted by force of habit.

Treating Hypoglycemia

- Be alert for early symptoms of hypoglycemia such as sweating, fast heartbeat, shaking, headache.
- Carry a source of sugar with you at all times. Hard candy, such as Life Savers, are easy to carry.
- Treat as soon as possible. Don't postpone therapy for any reason.
- If monitoring is not immediately available, treat and then check your blood sugar.
- The most rapid sources of sugar are liquids with sugar such as orange juice or soda (non-diet), or hard candies. Four to six ounces of soda or juice, or five Life Savers are usually sufficient.
- Repeat your therapy if symptoms aren't improving (or blood sugar isn't rising) within ten to fifteen minutes.
- Don't overtreat reactions. More sugar doesn't necessarily speed the rate of recovery from hypoglycemia, but will lead to subsequent elevated blood sugar levels.
- Make sure that family members, roommates, and fellow workers know how to treat you if you can't treat yourself. They should know how to give glucagon and to call an ambulance.
- Learn from each episode. Try to identify the cause of each one so you can prevent further occurrences.

Family, Friends, and Hypoglycemia

Your friends and relatives may be quite willing to tell you just how hard you were to deal with during your last hypoglycemic episode. They may even be tempted to blame you for your behavior, as though you deliberately became hypoglycemic to spite them. Several times, relatives of people under my treatment have groaned to me about how hard it was to "reason" with their spouse or child during hypoglycemia, and how this person had to be practically hit over the head to get some compliance. Unfortunately, frequent or severe hypoglycemia can become a major family problem, sometimes creating fear in children and friction between spouses.

Treating someone whose blood sugar is low can be a very frustrating experience. It's important for you, as a person with diabetes, to be aware of the effect your behavior during hypoglycemia can have on the individuals around you.

Sure, it's important to try to avoid hypoglycemia. *But the fact is that if you have IDDM and are trying to achieve tight blood sugar control, it is likely that you will have one or two hypoglycemic episodes a month.* However, with proper planning and preparation, you can make sure that most of them are mild and easily treated.

You need to let your family and friends know that hypoglycemia is part of your life. Make sure that they know you don't mean the things you say when you're hypoglycemic, and that you're not using hypoglycemia as an excuse to goof off or get attention. Tell them that you don't mean to react slowly or indifferently to them when your blood sugar is low. They need to know that this kind of behavior may be brought on by hypoglycemia.

Talking about hypoglycemia is a good way to introduce the larger issues of diabetes to people you know well, who may have misconceptions about your disease. They should understand that it's not the same as being under the influence of alcohol or drugs, and that if you are acting peculiarly or seem confused you may need their help.

An elderly patient once described to me a scene in which he begged some of his neighbors for sugar or candy, because he knew he was slipping into hypoglycemia. They stared back at him, paralyzed with fear.

"They thought that, since I was diabetic, I was addicted to sugar," he said angrily. "Can you believe that?"

Unfortunately, people have all kinds of wild ideas about diabetes. You should make it your business to let people know the truth about diabetes, particularly as it relates to hypoglycemia. It might save your life.

Here are some things that those who are close to you ought to know about hypoglycemia:

• The symptoms, listed previously, that indicate the onset.

• The easiest treatment is probably a sweet drink, like fruit juice, a nondiet soda, or even two to three teaspoons of sugar mixed into a glass of water. Skim milk may work, if nothing else is available.

• Smarties, Life Savers, or any kind of small sugary candy that is quickly digested, are good choices.

• People taking beta blockers for heart problems may not perceive the onset of hypoglycemia, because these drugs mask the warning effects of adrenaline.

• Recovery may be about fifteen minutes in coming.

• Don't put anything in the mouth of anyone who is unconscious.

• Glucagon, in the hands of someone who knows how to use it, may be extremely helpful (see next section).

• If you see someone who appears to be in hypoglycemia, don't panic. When in doubt, call an ambulance.

Glucagon

Hypoglycemia severe enough to preclude treatment with oral carbohydrate (decreased level of consciousness or inability to cooperate) should be treated either with an injection of glucagon (which all people with IDDM should have at home) or intravenously administered glucose (which you are unlikely to have at home). Like insulin, glucagon is a hormone, a substance naturally produced by the body that helps regulate glucose levels. However, glucagon has a function that opposes insulin: whereas insulin *reduces* the level of glucose in your blood, glucagon *increases* your blood sugar level. It does this by stimulating your liver to make and release glucose.

Glucagon effects this transformation extremely quickly, raising glucose levels in five to ten minutes. Because severe hypoglycemia is scary and glucagon is so effective at ending it, you will want it to be administered with a practiced hand, and without hesitation. But remember, you are not the one who will administer it! If you need glucagon, it is because you are incapable of treating yourself, most often because of altered consciousness. Someone else will need to know where it is and how to give it. Glucagon must be mixed *immediately* before use in order to be effective. The kits have a limited shelf life, so you need to remember to get a new prescription when the old vial expires. *If you have a hypoglycemic episode and need glucagon, there won't be time to call your doctor for a prescription and run to the pharmacy.* Keep an unexpired dose on hand; when it's expired, throw it out and replace it.

The procedure is really quite simple: the syringe comes loaded with a liquid that must be injected into the glucagon vial that comes with the kit. Once mixed, the vial should be shaken briefly to combine the two, and the mixture then drawn back into the syringe. The glucagon is now ready to be injected.

Glucagon injection follows the same general rules as a subcutaneous insulin injection. In an emergency situation, the skin does not need to be cleaned with alcohol. A small amount of skin should be pinched between thumb and forefinger, and the syringe inserted quickly. The glucagon is injected and the needle is withdrawn from the skin. Your physician or diabetes educator should review this technique with the people who are most likely to be with you when you need it, usually a parent, spouse, close friend, adult child, even a co-worker. There's no point in your knowing how to inject glucagon unless you use that knowledge to teach someone else. When you need it most, you are incapable of giving it to yourself. Family members and friends need to learn from you. Whoever is taught the technique should be reassured that they can't hurt you with glucagon. Not only is this true, but it will serve to relieve their anxiety about providing this very important first aid when it is necessary.

Troubleshooting Hypoglycemia

People who have lost their sensitivity to low blood sugar have to be extra careful about how they manage their diabetes. If you have difficulty identifying low blood sugars, here are some ideas for how to cope:

• First of all, keep track of when your low blood sugars occur. The timing of many low blood sugar events can be explained by the time of insulin peak action and daily schedules of meals and exercise. Working with your physician, nurse educator, or dietitian, you should be able to figure out which insulin dose or which behavior may be responsible for hypoglycemia, and thus need adjustment. Some reactions may occur during sleep—a potentially dangerous time to have a reaction, because it may not awaken you and may result in prolonged hypoglycemia. Testing blood sugar at 3 A.M. once every one to two weeks may help intensively treated IDDM patients find out if they're suffering from overnight lows.

• Monitor yourself more frequently. This can be a problem for people with busy jobs and lifestyles. However, new wipeless machines make it easier to monitor. People who monitor find it easier to stay in control, and if you monitor more often, you'll avoid hypoglycemia. You should always increase the frequency of your monitoring when you're sick with a cold or flu, when your exercise or eating schedules change, or when engaging in potentially dangerous activities. For instance, if you expect to drive a car for several hours, plan to check your blood sugar at least every couple of hours.

• Careful observations and recording of the events surrounding a hypoglycemic episode are key to identifying the specific causes of the event. Learn from the episode. Hypoglycemia should never be treated lightly.

Hypoglycemia in NIDDM

Insulin therapy can cause hypoglycemia in persons with NIDDM, just as in those with IDDM. But NIDDM patients appear to be much less likely to develop severe hypoglycemia, even when the treatment goal is to achieve normal glucose levels, compared with intensively treated patients with IDDM. This may be due to their resistance to insulin action, which serves to buffer them against inadvertent insulin overdosage. In addition, NIDDM patients don't appear to have the reduction in warning symptoms of hypoglycemia, which occurs so frequently in IDDM, and can lead to severe hypoglycemia.

On the other hand, even though hypoglycemia may be less frequent in insulin-treated NIDDM patients than in IDDM patients, *any* episode of hypoglycemia may be more dangerous in the NIDDM person. The increased risk associated with hypoglycemia lies in the older age of the NIDDM population and the more common occurrence of heart disease. Hypoglycemia results in a surge of adrenaline which may adversely affect anyone with heart disease.

NIDDM patients treated with diet alone or with diet and acarbose (Precose) or metformin (Glucophage) do not develop hypoglycemia. However, treatment with sulfonylureas (see Chapter 10) can cause hypoglycemia that may be quite severe. The episodes are more likely in patients with liver disease, or those who eat erratically or drink excessive alcohol. Unfortunately, many patients treated with anti-diabetic pills don't wear identification and may not be promptly identified as using hypoglycemic agents when found confused or admitted to an emergency room. This will delay emergency treatment. In addition, several of the available sulfonylureas have very long durations of action and can cause very long-lasting hypoglycemia. Therefore, patients with hypoglycemia caused by sulfonylureas often require admission to the hospital for prolonged observation and treatment.

Until new treatment methods have been developed, hypoglycemia will always be something that people treated with insulin or sulfonylureas have to live with. Do what you can to avoid it, try to prepare for it, but make these preparations with the goal of maintaining tight blood sugar control. In the next chapter, we'll talk about some of the possible consequences of failing to keep control of your blood sugar, and how to deal with those complications.

8

Complications of Diabetes

There is an old proverb that says, "I pay heed to my enemy; he teaches me patience." As mentioned in the Introduction, diabetes is a great teacher; it requires you to learn about your body, and, even more, about your strength as a person. But what diabetes can also teach is patience, because it has an unsurpassed ability to wait and wait and wait for its time to strike.

As most diabetologists can attest, caring for people with diabetes involves two major responsibilities. *First, care providers have to help patients learn to take care of themselves with regard to their metabolic or blood sugar control.* For most young, recent-onset IDDM patients, day-to-day sugar control, aimed at maintaining blood sugar levels as close to the nondiabetic range as possible, is their only self-care responsibility. They are otherwise generally healthy, and avoiding hypoglycemia and very high sugar levels is their first order of business. Long-term maintenance of near-normal sugar levels will do much to keep them healthy. Similarly, some patients with recent-onset NIDDM may also be generally healthy; however, given their older age and the associated obesity, hypertension, and abnormal lipids (cholesterol), NIDDM patients are more likely to have other health problems. Control of blood sugars is likely to be only one aspect of their overall care.

The second major component of providing care for people with diabetes is the never-ending vigilance for and treatment of its long-term complications. The detection of long-term complications, the attempts to prevent their development, and the treatment of those complications when they occur often monopolize the time and efforts of care providers and patients alike. The complications of diabetes are responsible for most of the suffering and the cost associated with the disease. Diabetes causes more cases of blindness, kidney failure, and amputations in adults than any other disease. In addition, it is a major contributor to heart disease. The total costs for diabetes care in the United States exceed $100 billion per year, and most of that cost is attributable to long-term complications.

The most awesome and fearful displays of the destructive power of diabetes don't occur overnight; they take place slowly, over time, insidiously gathering momentum until one day diabetes is more than an annoyance—it has become a major medical problem. This is the kind of patience diabetes has.

To help you understand why diabetes leaves you open to so many fearful complications, you may have to start thinking about the disease in a slightly different way. Diabetes is a disorder of *metabolism*, the process by which you regulate the energy you get from nourishment. In IDDM, this metabolic dysfunction is caused by a lack of insulin, whereas in NIDDM, it's caused by a combination of insulin resistance and insulin deficiency. Both these metabolic abnormalities lead to elevated blood sugar levels, as well as other abnormalities in fat and protein metabolism.

The other characteristic abnormality of all forms of diabetes is the development of disease in the body's small blood vessels, or *microvasculature,* and in the nervous system. Eyes, kidneys, and nerves are very vulnerable to diabetes. Everyone with diabetes—IDDM or NIDDM—is potentially vulnerable to its long-term complications. Because gestational diabetes (GDM) usually lasts for less than three or four months, it does not cause complications, unless the woman with GDM goes on to develop NIDDM.

Because you know that both high blood sugar levels and microvascular abnormalities are found in people with diabetes, you might naturally conclude that chronic exposure to the former causes the latter. Although the mechanism by which elevated blood sugar levels *cause* diabetic complications is unknown, there are several reasons why scientists think the two are closely related. First, in large studies of people with diabetes, the level of chronic blood sugar correlates with the development of complications. In other words, people with high blood sugar develop complications more frequently than people with better controlled blood sugar. Second, studies of animals with diabetes have shown that lowering blood sugar levels prevents complications. Finally, and most important, a recent landmark study in patients with IDDM, the Diabetes Control and Complications Trial

(DCCT), has demonstrated that maintaining lower blood sugar levels prevents the development of diabetic complications and slows their progression when they do occur. We'll learn more about all of the complications of diabetes and the results of the important DCCT in this chapter.

To avoid complications, you need to have more patience than diabetes, and that's a lot. You need the patience to deal with your disease every day: to monitor your blood sugar, regulate your diet, adjust your medication, and get regular exercise that will improve your circulation, your overall health, and give you the energy you need to cope with this disease. Your health care provider will need to perform special examinations to detect the development of these complications so that they can be treated aggressively if they develop. Diabetes will always be able to outwait you, so if you want to live a long time with this disease, and do it without severe complications, you will have to learn a lot of patience.

As you have read and will learn about in more detail in Chapter 11, the DCCT produced some very good news. Unlike many other people with chronic degenerative illnesses, you can do something about your problem. *You can drastically reduce your risk for all the long-term complications of diabetes with tighter blood sugar control. In the DCCT, this was achieved with intensive therapy in IDDM patients.* Although the DCCT studied only patients with IDDM, most experts agree that patients with NIDDM should benefit similarly from tight control of their blood sugar levels. The DCCT also suggested that *in some cases you can reverse or reduce the severity of complications with improved blood sugar control.* So that's why, throughout this book, I've stressed the importance of working with a diabetes treatment team to get your blood sugar under control.

Unfortunately, no matter how hard they try, some people with diabetes will develop complications. Many people can't control their blood sugar in the recommended range because it is hard to perform all the necessary tasks to achieve near-normal blood sugar control, or for other reasons. Some people may be more susceptible to the effects of diabetes for reasons that are not yet understood. Other factors can also come into play. For example, high blood pressure will make some complications more likely. Also, the longer you have diabetes, the more likely you are to develop complications. So, people who were diagnosed with diabetes at a very young age bear the greatest risk as they get older. Factors like these make it harder for some people to avoid complications.

If you have developed complications, or your doctor has told you that it looks likely that you will, don't give up on your self-treatment plan. In the past, most people with diabetes developed some evidence of complications; however, if they control their blood sugars, only a minority of patients will develop severe complications in the future. If you can keep your complications at a very mild stage, so much the better. Careful surveillance for the early stages of complications will allow your treatment team to limit their impact and preserve your health.

Even if complications have begun, you can continue to battle them with blood sugar control to reduce the risk of still more serious problems. In addition, careful attention to foot care, treatment of hypertension, and laser treatment for diabetic eye disease can all limit the damage caused by complications.

There are three major classes of diabetes-specific complications: retinopathy (eye disease), nephropathy (kidney disease), and neuropathy (nervous system complications). A less specific complication which can occur in nondiabetics but is markedly more common in diabetics is macrovascular disease (complications occurring in the large blood vessels, especially those supplying the heart, brain, and extremities). Combinations of these complications (neuropathy and peripheral vascular disease) make people with diabetes very susceptible to foot problems, which we'll discuss specifically at the end of the chapter. Each of the complications of diabetes can be extremely serious, and all deserve careful discussion. Let's start with a complication familiar to many people with diabetes, diabetic retinopathy.

Eye Disease

Shakespeare called the eyes "the windows of the soul." Indeed, they are perhaps, to the sighted, our most prized organ, for they allow us to experience and navigate our world in a way that other senses cannot. A person with diabetes who regained some of her lost sight with surgery once told me, "I feel that I'm living again."

The eye itself is a highly developed outgrowth of the brain. The principal light-sensing structures in the retina (the innermost layer of the eye) are rods and cones. These are designed to respond to light, transforming it into nerve impulses. These impulses are carried to the brain, where they are almost miraculously interpreted, providing a rich world of color, shade, definition, and movement that is instantaneously recorded and interpreted for our use.

Eye disease is one of the most common complications of diabetes, and diabetes is the most common cause of vision loss in adults in the United States. Early signs of retinopathy generally don't appear until five years after the diagnosis of IDDM. Children who have been diagnosed with diabetes may not display early signs of retinopathy until after puberty. Before the results of the DCCT were put into practice, studies indicated that by seven years after diagnosis, about half of patients with IDDM had some degree of retinopathy, usually mild. When people had IDDM for twenty years, their risk of suffering from some level of retinopathy rose to as high as 90 percent.

For people with NIDDM, the onset of diabetes is more insidious. NIDDM often goes undiagnosed for years after its onset. Since the early eye damage caused by diabetes is "silent," causing no symptoms, about 10 to 20 percent of people with NIDDM *already have eye disease at the time they're diagnosed with diabetes,* a sign that they have been in poor control of their blood sugar for some time.

The causes of retinopathy are not well understood, but the main events that take place have been well documented. There are two main stages in this process: *background retinopathy* and *proliferative retinopathy.* After the diagnosis of diabetes, changes start to take place in the microvasculature that nourishes the retina. Simply put, these small blood vessels become abnormal and leaky. The small blood vessel walls weaken, and small bubbles form, called *microaneurysms.* These microaneurysms leak red blood cells into the retina *(hemorrhages).* Shortly after, serum, the fluid in which blood cells circulate, escapes from these abnormal vessels, forming puddles within the multilayered retina. When the fluid is reabsorbed, the proteins and fats that were in the serum remain behind, leaving a white substance called a "hard exudate." The formation of microaneurysms, hemorrhages, and exudates is called *background*, or *nonproliferative*, retinopathy.

When circulation to the retina is decreased, a different type of exudate begins to form, called a *soft exudate*, or *cotton wool spot*. A more advanced form of nonproliferative retinopathy, these abnormalities represent the deterioration of nerve fibers in the retina resulting from the lack of oxygen. In general, the nonproliferative retinopathy we have described so far doesn't usually affect vision. However, if leakage of fluid occurs near the *macula* (a part of the retina that provides much of our visual acuity), it can result in a condition called *macular edema*, which makes vision much less sharp.

With more extensive blockage of blood supply to the retina, the eye responds by forming new blood vessels. While this sounds like a protective response, the formation of these new vessels, called proliferative retinopathy, can lead to severe eye problems.

"These new blood vessels are not worth the trouble of making them," says Dr. Mara Lorenzi, an investigator at Mass General who studies the effect of diabetes on blood vessels. "They leak, break easily, and release blood and fluids into the eye, stimulating more inappropriate new vessel formation."

When one of the new vessels bleeds, a relatively large amount of blood is released, sometimes blocking vision suddenly and frighteningly. Although the blood usually clears itself in several weeks to months, and vision clears, more problems occur as the eye reacts to the proteins and fluids that have escaped into the retina.

Immune cells migrate to the site of the bleeding, responding as they always do to an injury. They release factors that promote more blood vessel growth and, later, scarring. Such scarring can have a profound effect on vision. When the scar shrinks, the retina may detach from the back of the eye. The detachment causes severe loss of vision that is often permanent.

Diagnosis

The earlier that retinopathy is detected, the more likely it is that loss of vision can be prevented or slowed. This is why it's extremely important to have your eyes checked regularly. Annual eye exams with an eye specialist are recommended after five years of IDDM, and from the time of diagnosis with NIDDM. Studies have shown that only about half the people with diabetes get the eye care they need, including yearly examinations for retinopathy. If retinopathy is caught and treated early enough, vision can be preserved for quite some time. If, on the other hand, retinopathy is allowed to progress without treatment, vision loss may occur, sometimes irreversibly. I asked Mara Lorenzi to give some perspective on diagnosing diabetic retinopathy.

"During background retinopathy, we can see typical abnormalities in the small vessels of the retina. These trouble spots can be viewed using an *ophthalmoscope,* the small tool you probably remember your doctor using to look into your eye. Adults with diabetes should have a dilated-eye examination at least once a year. This is particularly important for diabetic women during pregnancy, when retinopathy can worsen rapidly. When your eyes are dilated, they will be very sensitive to light for a few hours, so remember to bring sunglasses. You will also have difficulty focusing and will need to take public transportation, or have a friend or relative drive you. These effects of dilation usually last for three to four hours.

"In cases where a more sensitive tool is needed, *stereoscopic fundus photography* is performed. This is a sophisticated method of photographing the retina that allows your doctor to see damage to the eye in great detail. Another diagnostic technique is *fluorescein angiography*, in which a small amount of dye is injected into the bloodstream, making the blood vessels in the eye much more visible for diagnosis. The dye itself makes some people nauseous, but this usually disappears quickly. The dye also turns your urine orange for a few days, which can be rather frightening if you are not prepared for it, but it's harmless.

"When we see dots of broken blood vessels and yellowish material in the surrounding tissue, that means that blood vessels have become permeable and are leaking into the surrounding tissue. Now, often this will take place and no vision problems will occur, but when the same rate of leakage occurs near the maculae they will begin to detect changes in vision.

"If macular edema develops, this could mean a severe vision problem, because the macula is the part of the retina that gives us our visual acuity. If you develop edema, the macula is no longer capable of giving you precise images, and you have some visual loss. Macular edema is often first detected when vision becomes so blurry that a person can no longer distinguish objects from one another.

Treatment

Make no mistake; the best treatment for diabetic eye disease is *prevention*. If you don't have eye disease now, keeping your blood sugar under control, as demonstrated by the DCCT, can help you avoid significant retinopathy for years. In addition, blood sugar control in the near-normal range slows the progression of existing nonproliferative retinopathy. Once background (nonproliferative) retinopathy progresses to proliferative retinopathy, tight blood sugar control may no longer be counted on to prevent worsening of the condition.

Fortunately, we live in an era in which treatment for the more severe stages of diabetic eye disease has improved greatly. The most common form of treatment is *photocoagulation*, or laser therapy. Laser therapy can help reduce macular edema and proliferative retinopathy. The purpose of this treatment in macular edema is to "dry out" the eye by closing off the leaking vessels, usually with a small number of laser burns.

When proliferative retinopathy is present, a large number of burns are made with the goal of destroying parts of the retina that are not crucial for vision, but which are using oxygen. By burning part of the retina, the stimulus for new vessel growth is eliminated and the fragile new vessels shrink. This strategy is effective in preventing further bleeding and loss of vision. Laser treatment comes with a price, however; the peripheral retina that is used for night vision and to provide full visual fields is destroyed. When this tissue is destroyed with laser therapy, vision at night may suffer and your peripheral vision may decrease.

In 1980, Gail Denman was a twenty-one-year-old senior at a Pennsylvania college, teaching first grade through an internship. An energetic, sociable woman who enjoys talking and joking, she loved her work and was only slightly worried when she found that she was having a little trouble seeing. She noticed that there were little black spots, or "floaters," in her field of vision. She had no idea what it meant. Then, one day she looked up at the blackboard directly behind her and realized that she couldn't see what was written on it, even with her glasses. She realized that it was time to see an ophthalmologist.

For Gail, diagnosis with proliferative retinopathy was a horrifying, mystifying experience. After the brief examination, she recalls, her doctor looked directly at her and said to her, "You are going blind. You are going to lose all your vision." She immediately returned home to the Boston area to seek treatment.

Laser treatment for eye disease is effective, but it can sometimes be painful. Unfortunately, Gail was one of the minority for whom it was painful. When Gail described her experiences to me, which she still recalls in great detail, her normally lighthearted tone became much more grave.

"I underwent panretinal photocoagulation every two or three weeks for three months, from October to December of 1980. I probably had a total of about five treatments. Each treatment probably involved about 200 burns in each eye, so there were about a thousand burns in each eye.

"It was very painful. My eyes hurt, and I just felt a great deal of constant anxiety, knowing each time that I was going to have to sit with my head held still. The laser was this green beam that went right into my eye! Tears would come streaming down. Somehow, I had to get through it, and I did. It saved my vision.

"I had to keep little patches over my eyes for five days after each treatment. And I had to lie flat, because we didn't want blood moving around while the burns were healing. If I sat up too quick, another hemorrhage might have hit. I still can't lift heavy things, because any kind of high pressure in my eyes might cause a hemorrhage. I remember once when, during treatment, I saw a hemorrhage inside my eye. It was as if someone had taken red and black spray paint and sprayed it inside my eye.

"You have to slow yourself down in some ways. Swimming can be a problem. I had a hemorrhage a few years ago when, stupidly, I dove into the water. It's too bad because my husband Jim is a diver, and of course I can't do anything like that. He goes every week. He gave me a diving pendant to keep me happy."

Gail also suffers from a fairly common complication of diabetes, diabetic cataract. A cataract is a small opacity or cloud that appears in the lens of the eye. Some scientists suspect that formation of these cataracts could also be linked to poor blood sugar control. Gail recently underwent surgical removal of her cataracts, which has restored a great deal of the vision she had lost over the past ten years, since the cataracts began developing.

"I feel like I'm living my life all over again," she told me, just a couple of days after her surgery. "We just moved into this house in September, and I never really saw it then. Now I feel like I'm seeing it for the first time. After the surgery, I looked at Jim and said, 'You need a haircut.' "

Still, Gail is legally blind, meaning that she can see things clearly with glasses at 20 feet that people with normal vision can see clearly at 200 feet. Although she can still see and even read—using extremely high-powered glasses—her condition has had a profound impact on her life. The support she gets from her husband and her parents is crucial to her ability to cope with diabetic eye disease.

When Gail was single, she lived on Boston's Beacon Hill, within walking distance to her office at the Massachusetts Commission for the Blind, where she now works. Now that she and Jim have moved back to the suburb of Weston, where Gail grew up, they found a house adjacent to a commuter rail station. This makes Gail's daily travel to and from work safer and simpler.

Fortunately, Gail has a long history of support from family members. Her mother, who also has IDDM, diagnosed Gail at the age of nine during a family vacation in Canada. This was the beginning of many health difficulties they've been through together. Gail talks about her relationship with her mother frequently and gratefully.

"My mom took me to every one of my treatments. My mom's a wonderful lady. She's sixty-one and has never suffered any complications of diabetes that I know of, except that she occasionally has had low blood sugars that have resulted in some pretty serious near misses with the car." Gail laughed at the thought but then became serious again.

"I think my mother feels guilty, but that hasn't stopped her from being there every step of the way."

I asked Gail how she knew that her mother felt responsible for the suffering she's endured from eye disease.

"She doesn't express it verbally as much as I see it and feel it. Ever since she diagnosed me in the middle of the night, I've been able to tell that she's been uncomfortable about the idea of my having diabetes. Then I start feeling uncomfortable because she does. She'll talk about it sometimes, but she hates to see me in pain. She feels responsible, and she really shouldn't. Both my parents have said to me at different times, 'I wish I had these vision problems instead of you.' "

Gail's story represents the "dark side" of the diabetes force. She grew up with diabetes in a period before the importance of tight blood sugar control was recognized and before intensive therapy methods to achieve those goals were available. Although laser therapy preserved her vision, she is left with a significant deficit. We now know that most of the problems she experienced can be prevented, and far fewer people with IDDM and NIDDM will need laser treatment or lose their vision in the future.

Kidney Disease

Kidney disease is a common and serious complication of diabetes, perhaps the most serious, developing in about 35 percent of people with IDDM and 10 to 15 percent of people with NIDDM. The most serious stage of kidney disease results in *end-stage renal failure,* a life-threatening condition that, while treatable with dialysis or transplantation, is extremely debilitating and frequently fatal. Diabetes is the most common cause of renal failure, which causes a total of more than 60,000 deaths each year.

The kidneys serve a very important purpose: they filter toxins and waste from your bloodstream, excreting them in urine. The kidneys also play a critical role in regulating the amount of salt and water in your body, which affects weight and blood pressure. They also help determine how many red blood cells are made by your bone marrow, and they regulate bone formation by promoting the production of a potent form of vitamin D. Obviously, kidneys are extremely complex organs, and when they begin to fail, many bodily functions suffer.

The kidney's filtering process is mainly performed in small structures called *glomeruli*. Each *glomerulus* is a delicate lattice of tiny blood vessels and tubules. Waste water, toxins, and other unnecessary or harmful substances are transported from the blood, across these membranes, and into the tubules and then they are directed out of the kidney to the bladder for excretion. The kidney filters a tremendous amount of blood, more than a quart every *minute*.

The glomeruli and blood vessels in the kidney are sensitive to the changes that take place during diabetes. Not long after the onset of diabetes, microscopic changes begin to occur in the glomeruli, all of which are related to long-term kidney damage:

1. A few months after diagnosis, the rate of filtration within the glomerulus increases in about 30 to 40 percent of people with diabetes. Some studies have suggested that this increased blood filtration may be harmful, causing stress to the glomeruli. Tight blood sugar control can bring the glomerular filtration rate back down into the normal range.

2. While glomerular filtration rate increases, kidney enlargement, or *nephromegaly*, may occur. The kidneys can increase to one-and-a-half times their normal size.

3. Three to five years after the onset of diabetes, increased amounts of small proteins, which are usually

retained by the kidney, begin to leak into the urine. The major protein in the urine is albumin. Usually only very small quantities of albumin, less than 20 milligrams per day, appear in the urine. However, as microscopic changes progress in the diabetic kidney, increasing quantities of albumin leak through the glomerulus and appear in the urine. This early stage of renal dysfunction, called *microalbuminuria,* is usually measured most accurately in a 12- or 24-hour urine collection. Microalbuminuria is a long-term predictor of kidney disease. The majority of people with IDDM who develop microalbuminuria ultimately go on to develop increased albumin excretion, called *clinical albuminuria,* which can be detected easily with a simple dipstick test. (The significance of albuminuria in NIDDM is not as clear.) The progression from microalbuminuria to clinical albuminuria usually takes longer than ten years. More than 90 percent of patients with clinical albuminuria unfortunately go on to develop severe kidney disease, a process that takes another five to ten years. During this final phase, the filtering and other functions of the kidney begin to fail.

As the glomerular filtration rate starts to drop off in the late stages of kidney disease, a number of problems develop. Because the kidney can't handle water and salt as it used to and because of the protein loss in the urine, swelling (or *edema*) occurs, usually in the feet, but sometimes in the hands, too. If you have edema, you may notice increasing swelling in your feet and ankles later in the day, and facial swelling in the morning when you've just awakened. In addition, you may begin to develop anemia (low blood count) and bone thinning, a form of osteoporosis. Also, high blood pressure almost always accompanies the worsening of kidney function. Fortunately, all of these problems can be treated, if they are recognized. Treatment of high blood pressure is especially important, because it can further damage the kidney. As if all of the above weren't severe enough, large-blood-vessel disease, including blockage of the blood vessels supplying the heart and legs, speeds up in people with kidney failure.

The film *Steel Magnolias* portrayed, in dramatic Hollywood fashion, the horror of diabetic kidney disease. A young woman who suffers from IDDM dies rather suddenly of kidney disease not long after having given birth to her first child. The portrayal is heartrending, but not very realistic. The time span from the beginning of diabetes to the development of end-stage disease, which requires dialysis or transplantation, is usually more than twenty years. Moreover, research has demonstrated opportunities for treatment to slow the progress of kidney disease at almost every step of the way. People who keep regular appointments with their diabetologist or kidney specialist usually get good advice on how to take care of their kidneys and forestall end-stage renal failure as long as possible.

When scarring of the kidney becomes more severe, the waste and poisons that the kidneys normally filter out begin to build up, and obvious symptoms of kidney disease may appear. These can include confusion, fatigue, nausea, shortness of breath, and itching. As the prospect of end-stage renal failure looms, people with kidney disease must consider treatment with either dialysis or kidney transplantation. Chemical changes such as an elevated potassium level, uncontrollable edema, or the symptoms noted above often signal the need for dialysis.

In the past, there was seemingly no way to prevent the loss of kidney function and progression toward end-stage renal failure. Because of the DCCT, however, we now have evidence that tight blood sugar control can indeed play a role in preventing or slowing the progress of nephropathy. At the same time, recently completed studies show that treatments that lower blood pressure also hold new hope for slowing the progression of kidney diseases. Remember, even before these new therapies were available, only 35 percent of IDDM patients and 10 to 15 percent of NIDDM patients developed kidney disease. Now even fewer diabetic patients will have to face dialysis or transplantation because of end-stage kidney disease.

Diagnosis

As we've seen, kidney disease is an extremely serious health problem that can result in severe disability or even death. It's very important to keep an eye on your kidneys and blood pressure, and make sure that your physician does, too.

As mentioned, the first measurable sign of kidney disease is usually elevated albumin excretion. Normally, the amount of albumin in your urine should be less than 20 milligrams every 24 hours. If your doctor sees a urine albumin level that is repeatedly above 20 mg/24 hours, he or she will begin to take early, precautionary treatment measures. At some point, you may be referred to a kidney specialist, or *nephrologist,* for further treatment.

Your doctor may suggest that you provide either a random, or "spot," urine test, or a 24-hour urine sample to look for these problems. Although a 24-hour urine collection is inconvenient (you need to urinate into a clean collection jug, which your doctor or laboratory will supply, for an entire 24-hour cycle), it is the best method to diagnose kidney problems definitively, especially in their early stages. So even though you may need to explain why you are lugging around a brown jug—which you should label, "This is not apple juice!!!" when you put it in the refrigerator—the payoff of reassuring yourself or discovering the problem early enough to provide effective treatment should make up for any minor embarrassment. I usually tell my patients to try to pick a convenient day when they are not exercising vigorously or traveling. In addition, if they have any symptoms suggestive of a urinary tract infection—a burning sensation with urination, for example—they should postpone the collection until their symptoms are treated. On the morning of the collection,

---

How to Collect a 24-Hour Urine Sample

- Select a day when you can conveniently perform the collection.
- No vigorous exercise on the two days before and the day of the collection.
- If you have symptoms of a possible bladder infection (burning sensation with urination or cloudy urine), postpone the collection and call your physician.
- The first urine on the morning of the collection goes into the toilet.
- All subsequent urine (every drop) goes into the collection jug, including the first urine in the morning of the second day.
- Store urine jug (appropriately labeled!) in the refrigerator until you bring it to the laboratory—within forty-eight hours.

urinate into the toilet when you first wake up. All subsequent urine should be collected in the jug, including the first urine of the next morning. To make collecting the urine easier for women, the laboratory can supply a special receptacle to place in the toilet.

Under normal circumstances, your doctor may ask for a 24-hour urine collection and a blood test to measure the level of creatinine (a waste substance that the kidney usually excretes and that increases if the kidney is beginning to fail) on a yearly to every-other-year basis, depending on how long you have had your diabetes. However, if your kidney abnormalities begin to progress, you may have more frequent monitoring. Your doctor may also check the blood protein levels, the clearance rate of creatinine, and other indicators of the bone disease and anemia that can potentially accompany kidney disease. Your physician may warn you to avoid certain commonly used anti-inflammatory drugs, called *nonsteroidal anti-inflammatory drugs* or *NSAIDs,* such as ibuprofen. You may also receive warnings against receiving dyes as part of x-ray procedures, because of their potential effect on the kidneys.

Treatment

The first step in taking care of kidney disease is to maintain tight blood sugar control. As we'll see in Chapter 11, the DCCT showed that tight blood sugar control results in a 39 percent lower risk of developing microalbuminuria and a more than 50 percent reduction in developing even more advanced stages of kidney disease.

High blood pressure has also been implicated in hastening the course of kidney disease. Effective therapy slows the rate of kidney failure in the later stages. Although most, but not all, drugs that lower blood pressure have a similar beneficial effect on kidney disease, one particular class of antihypertensive drug seems to have an additional benefit, both in the early and later stages.

Recent studies of people with IDDM and NIDDM have demonstrated that the angiotensin-converting enzyme inhibitors (ACE inhibitors) can lower the rate of kidney disease at the early stages when microalbuminuria is detectable, when patients have even higher levels of albumin excretion, and even later on when they have decreasing glomerular filtration. Although very long term studies have not been done, most experts are convinced that improving the early stages of kidney disease will inevitably slow its progression and perhaps decrease the occurrence of the more severe stages. There are a variety of ACE inhibitors available, and they are usually well tolerated with few side effects. The most common side effect is the development of a dry, intermittent cough, which occurs in no more than 10 percent of patients. Although the cough can be irritating, many patients find it only a minor inconvenience and "learn to live with it."

Still, intensive diabetes therapy and ACE inhibitors only slow kidney disease progression; they probably can't stop it. For people who do progress to end-stage renal failure (once a death sentence), there are now two lifesaving options. The first is dialysis, the filtering of toxins and fluid from the body. There are two kinds of dialysis, *hemodialysis* and *peritoneal dialysis*. Peritoneal dialysis, which involves administering several quarts of fluid through a small plastic tube or catheter into the abdominal chamber and then draining it, can be performed at home. Hemodialysis is usually performed at a treatment facility, because it involves filtering the blood through a complex artificial kidney. Almost anyone who has undergone dialysis can tell you that it is a difficult and time-consuming treatment.

After losing all her kidney function, as well as her sight, Pamela Martin underwent hemodialysis for three years. Four times a week, she went to a nearby hospital for four hours of treatment. Like many dialysis patients, she found it to be a very hard life.

"Your whole body breaks down," she recalls. "You're tired, you want to do lots of stuff but your body won't get up and go. Your mind becomes frustrated because you don't have any strength. It's a job, a full-time job."

Several quarts of water may be removed from your body during dialysis. This can leave you with drastically lowered blood pressure, and you may feel a bit woozy and sluggish. People who are on dialysis are urged to maintain a low-protein diet, and restrict their fluid and salt intake. However, many dialysis patients fail to follow their diets because they feel frustrated and discouraged.

Because of the frequency of treatment, it's hard to plan any kind of travel. "One time I wanted to go to Canada," recalls Pamela, a Micmac Indian woman who grew up on a reservation in northern Ontario. "I waited until after my treatment on Friday and had to be back early on Monday. I remember them telling me, 'Make sure that you're back on Monday,' because there's no telling what would have happened if I hadn't been. And all the time I was gone, I had to avoid drinking, drinking anything. 'Just breathe the air,' they told me. So for two days I lived on ice cubes, and that was hard. There are a lot of things you have to sacrifice."

An alternative therapy for diabetic patients with end-stage renal disease is transplantation. It is often the first choice, especially for younger people for whom the quality of life after a transplant is better than with dialysis. Unfortunately, the availability of donor kidneys is very limited, and patients often have to wait as long as two years, or even longer, for an appropriate kidney.

Two years ago, after three years of dialysis, Pamela was fortunate enough to receive a kidney transplant. Kidney transplantation, which originated in the 1950s at what was then Boston's Peter Bent Brigham Hospital, is perhaps the most advanced of all transplant procedures. According to Dr. Hugh Auchincloss, a transplant surgeon at Mass General, almost nine out of ten people who undergo kidney transplants have a functioning transplant for at least a year after the operation. More and more diabetic patients at Mass General have had functioning kidney transplants for more than ten years. However, the transplant options for people over fifty years of age are limited, because transplantable kidneys are in short supply and allocated partially on the basis of who stands to benefit most from them.

Taking an internal organ from one human being and transplanting it into another is extremely difficult and complex. The complexity doesn't stop with the surgery, either. As Dr. Auchincloss points out, surgeons follow the people in whom they've put new organs for the rest of their lives. "It's an interesting paradox," he says, "because we're thought of as very specialized surgeons, and yet for our patients we really become something like a primary care provider. I'm involved in almost every health decision my patients make."

The success of an organ transplant is determined in large part by the quality of the "match" between the organ and its new host. The body's immune system normally repels invaders of all kinds; if a new kidney were to appear inside you overnight, your immune system would assume that it was up to no good and immediately start trying to reject it. Rejection is an all-out immune attack on the transplanted organ; it's just as if the new organ were an infection, and your body was trying to fight it off.

There are a number of drugs that blunt this attack on your immune system, thereby allowing your body to hold on to the transplanted organ longer. The names of some of these drugs are *cyclosporine, imuran,* and *prednisone,* and as a class they are known as *immunosuppressants,* because they suppress your immune system. Prednisone is a relatively common steroid that you may have taken briefly if you've ever had poison ivy. While these drugs are generally safe in the short term, their long-term effects can be much harder to bear. Steroids cause weight gain and bone demineralization; cyclosporine causes high blood pressure and, paradoxically, kidney damage. They all predispose transplant patients to a variety of infections.

"The worst thing that can happen as a result of long-term cyclosporine is lymphoma, or cancer of the lymph glands," says Dr. Auchincloss. "The number of patients that develop lymphoma is directly related to how much cyclosporine they receive. If you give them more cyclosporine, they are less likely to undergo organ rejection, but they are more likely to get lymphoma. Therefore, regulating the dosage is always a delicate and unpredictable balance."

If the match is good, then the body is more likely to accept the new organ without much of a fuss. Guy Pollard is a technician from the Massachusetts Institute of Technology, right across the river from Mass General. He has had IDDM since his teen years, and five years ago, at the age of thirty-eight and after twenty-six years of diabetes, his kidneys failed. Luckily his sister's immune profile matched his perfectly (this is often called an *HLA match*) and she was willing to donate a kidney to Guy.

"The new kidney is fabulous," Guy says. "I had the transplant in 1991, and have never had a sign of rejection. The only problem has been that swings in my creatinine level affect my need for insulin, and I've had some bouts of hypoglycemia. I solved that by taking six or seven smaller injections of insulin each day and monitoring frequently. It's worked out just fine. I've got my blood sugar under good control, and it's been very liberating."

Some patients, on the other hand, do not match as well with the kidneys transplanted into them. Every few weeks, Patty Hall and her mother drive down from a small town in New Hampshire to see Dr. Auchincloss and talk to him about her third transplanted kidney. She represents the other extreme: her body has rejected two kidneys in the past year and she is now hoping that her third kidney will "take."

Two years ago, Patty's kidneys were failing and she was looking at the prospects of dialysis or transplantation. She knew that the root cause of her kidney disease was diabetes and decided that, if the possibility arose, she would undergo a pancreas transplant along with the kidney transplant. Mass General was among the early hospitals doing combined transplants, offering them to suitable diabetes patients because the pancreas transplant can essentially cure diabetes, relieving the need for insulin injections.

"I lost the kidney and the pancreas transplants, and I was really sick for a long time," Patty recalls. "I came back in and got a transplant from my sister and that lasted all of twenty-four hours. [This was one of only two combined kidney and pancreas transplants done at Mass General in the last six years that didn't take.] I finally got my third kidney, and while that has worked out okay, I've had a stroke and then open-heart surgery. And here I am today."

Most people who have been on dialysis for any length of time see the receipt of a new kidney as a chance for a new life, and indeed it is. However, the kidney is not the only organ that deteriorates in people with diabetes. Many patients with advanced kidney disease have needed laser treatments or have lost vision, and they may have serious neuropathy and sometimes heart disease by the time they receive a new kidney. The severity of these complications emphasizes the need to prevent their development with tight blood sugar control.

Neuropathy

Diabetic neuropathy has many manifestations: it can affect the sensory nerves (those that give us information about our environment, such as hot and cold), the motor nerves that move our muscles, or the autonomic nerves that control such functions as breathing and heartbeat. The most common clinical form of diabetic neuropathy affects the long sensory and motor nerves that emerge from the spine and travel to the feet or hands. People who have had diabetes for more than five years often report feeling a sensation of numbness or tingling that starts in the toes or fingers and slowly progresses to involve the feet, ankles, and sometimes even the lower legs. The abnormal sensation is sometimes described as "feeling as if I'm walking on cotton," "as if there's something between my sock and shoe," or "as if my feet are asleep." Although neuropathy is generally not too unpleasant, some people may develop painful symptoms that are sharp, shooting, or burning. These more severe symptoms are, thankfully, quite rare, but when they occur, they can interfere with sleep and require medication.

Usually, the sensory symptoms affect both sides similarly and are worse at night. Although many people assume and fear that a problem with circulation is causing the symptoms, I try to reassure them that neuropathy is usually only minimally bothersome and, with good foot care, won't cause significant problems. Symptoms of blood vessel blockage usually get worse with activity, whereas those of neuropathy improve.

More than one half of all diabetic patients will develop some evidence of peripheral sensory neuropathy, so don't be surprised if your doctor tests your ankle reflexes or vibration sensation with a tuning fork and tells you that you have neuropathy. As with all long-term diabetic complications, sensory neuropathy is more likely to develop after you have had diabetes for some time. It affects patients with both IDDM and NIDDM. Interestingly, many patients say that their neuropathy improves and becomes less noticeable over time. What has really happened is that the nerve abnormalities have gotten worse. With partial function of the nerves early in the course of neuropathy, patients receive funny messages from the nerves, which explains the "pins and needles" sensation. As nerve function worsens, these abnormal sensations decrease, but the feet are left with less feeling. When the nerve abnormality is particularly severe, people have difficulty feeling any sensations. I have had patients come into the office with thumbtacks or insulin needles stuck in their feet, and they don't feel a thing! You can well imagine how risky this is. The amount of time we spend on our feet and the pressure we place on them is something most of us take for granted. In people who have diabetic neuropathy, any minor trauma to the feet, such as chafing from a new pair of shoes that are a little tight, can lead to a calamity. With diminished sensation, you don't respond in the usual way, which would be to take the shoes off. Instead, you may wear the shoes all day, only to discover a blister or ulceration (hole) where they have literally worn away the skin. If the ulcer becomes infected or if circulation to your feet is poor, healing can be slow, if it occurs at all. Such "neuropathic" ulcers are the major cause of amputations in people with diabetes. With good foot care, most of these problems can be avoided (see the last section in this chapter).

There are other, less common forms of diabetic neuropathy. Whereas peripheral sensory neuropathy, described above, is a systematic problem, probably caused by the long-term effects of elevated glucose on long nerves, there are other forms of neuropathy that affect specific nerves and muscles. Such neuropathy is usually sudden and painless, and it causes weakness in a single group of muscles. Facial, arm, or leg muscles are most commonly affected, but there may also be weakness in muscles that control eye movement. Double vision, hand weakness, or foot drop (inability to move a foot upwards) can all be caused by this form of neuropathy. These motor neuropathies are thought to be caused by the obstruction (blockage) of individual small blood vessels that supply particular nerves. With decreased blood supply, the nerves are injured. Happily, the vast majority of these neuropathies, called *focal neuropathies,* recover by themselves over a period of six weeks to six months. So even though you may need a cane or foot brace for temporary assistance, don't despair—it will probably get better.

The other area of the nervous system that is affected by diabetes is the autonomic nervous system. As I noted earlier, this part of the nervous system responds automatically to regulate heartbeat, blood pressure, stomach and intestinal activity, urination, sexual function, and other self-regulating functions, even sweating. When the autonomic nervous system is affected, you may experience subtle changes, which only your doctor may notice, or more severe symptoms may occur. For example, your doctor may observe that your resting heart rate is faster than it used to be. On the other hand, you may notice that you become dizzy or light-headed if you sit up too quickly. Other forms of autonomic neuropathy can affect the stomach, causing a sense of fullness or discomfort after eating only a few bites of food; damage to nerves controlling the lower intestines may lead to alternating patterns of diarrhea, especially at night, and constipation; damage to bladder nerves may cause a pattern of frequent urination with small quantities, or even incontinence; and sexual dysfunction with impotence in men can also occur. Most of these complications affect no more than 10 to 20 percent of people with diabetes, although impotence may occur in as many as 50 percent of men with long-term diabetes.

There are reasonably effective treatments for all these autonomic neuropathy symptoms. Unfortunately, when these problems occur, they can affect other features of diabetes care. For example, slowed stomach activity, or *gastroparesis* as it's called, can interfere with absorption of nutrients and contribute to unstable blood sugar control. In addition, altered sweating patterns will predispose patients to develop dry, cracked skin, which makes good foot care even more difficult.

Diagnosis

Nerves are the body's information superhighway. They transmit messages from one area to another (for example, from the feet to the brain, and vice versa) using electrical impulses that communicate almost instantaneously. Quick transfer of information is an essential part of our nervous system.

Tests called *nerve conduction studies* measure how fast nerve impulses travel. In these studies, sensors that measure electrical activity in very small areas are attached to your arms, fingers, legs, or toes. Then specific nerves are stimulated and the speed of transmission is measured. This tells your doctor how well your nerves conduct their signals. Although most neuropathies are diagnosed when your doctor takes your medical history and examines you, nerve conduction studies may help him or her determine whether you have a sensory or focal motor neuropathy.

It doesn't usually take sophisticated tests to diagnose most diabetic neuropathies. Patients usually tell us what's wrong: they may feel pain, they may not be able to feel their feet, or they may have trouble with impotence. People with gastroparesis are usually diagnosed by an early sense of fullness after eating, abdominal discomfort, vomiting, or nausea.

However, sometimes the symptoms of autonomic neuropathy are not so clear, and specific tests must be performed. In order to evaluate gastroparesis, a meal study is often performed. In these studies, you'll eat a regular meal containing a tiny amount of radioactivity, and the movement of the food out of your stomach is monitored. If the emptying of your stomach is delayed, you'll be diagnosed with gastroparesis. Similarly, damage to bladder nerves can lead to ineffective bladder emptying, resulting in incontinence or recurrent bladder and kidney infections. In order to diagnose the cause, your doctor will measure the ability of your bladder to contract and empty. These studies may be performed by a *urologist,* who specializes in problems of the urinary tract.

As mentioned, the most common neuropathy may result in insensitivity of your feet and place them at risk, even during usual daily activities like walking. If you take your feet for granted, you may be in for real problems. That's why the most important part of diabetic foot care is your own management program. If you have diabetes, you should inspect your feet daily, looking for any signs of rubbing, blisters, or redness. You should be instructed in proper care of toenails, calluses, and corns. You are the first line of defense: look for cuts and sores that won't heal and report anything unusual to your doctor or podiatrist. We'll talk more about this in the last section of this chapter.

Glucose Control

As we've seen from the DCCT, people who want to reduce their chances of complications can do so by keeping their blood sugars as close to normal as possible. The same benefit is seen for the peripheral and autonomic neuropathies. In Chapter 11, you can see in more detail the dramatic difference that tight blood sugar control makes in the development of nerve damage.

However, once nerve damage has set in, it's not clear

how much can be done. Thus, prevention remains the best choice for combating neuropathy.

There are some specific treatments for the symptoms of diabetic neuropathy:

- Sensory neuropathy. A number of oral medications and creams can be used to alleviate painful symptoms, if they occur. None of these is uniformly effective and all have side effects. If you have sensory neuropathy, a realistic goal should be to relieve your symptoms at night so you can get a good night's sleep. You, and your doctor, should try to avoid using narcotics in this situation, unless absolutely necessary, because the risk of addiction is high. Painful neuropathy is often intermittent—the challenge is to get through the difficult time and achieve a good quality of life.

- Motor neuropathy. As I noted earlier, although the effects of a motor neuropathy may be disabling, they are usually only temporary. Using an eye patch to stop double vision or an ankle brace to counteract foot drop may be necessary, but usually only for several weeks or months. Another type of focal neuropathy that is common in diabetes is *compression neuropathy*. The most common example is carpal tunnel syndrome, which occurs when one of the large nerves in the wrist becomes compressed by the fibrous tunnels through which it travels. The compression causes numbness of the first three fingers and weakness in the thumb. These compression neuropathies, sometimes called *entrapment syndromes,* occur because diabetic nerves are relatively sensitive to pressure and because the tunnels through which they travel are narrower. Nerve conduction studies are necessary to diagnose the level of obstruction. If you have compression neuropathies, your doctor may recommend hand splints to decrease painful symptoms, but surgery is often necessary to release the nerve from its tight confines.

• Gastrointestinal problems. Gastroparesis symptoms can be relieved with two drugs, Reglan or Propulsid, that increase stomach contraction. Changes in diet sometimes help, but not reliably. Diabetic diarrhea and constipation can often be treated by increasing fiber in the diet, either with high-fiber foods or with fiber supplements, such as Metamucil. For more severe diarrhea, your doctor may try other drugs, including Clonidine, Imodium, or Lomotil, even an old-fashioned medicine called tincture of opium.

• Impotence. There are several approaches to treating impotence caused by diabetes. Vacuum devices can be used to help achieve erection. In addition, several drugs directly injected into the penis can be used to achieve an erection. Finally, specialized devices that help achieve erections can be surgically implanted. These devices, which are virtually undetectable, are very effective in restoring sexual function with a high level of satisfaction for men and their partners. Treatment of impotence can be complicated and often requires consultation with a urologist. However, with therapy men are often able to resume fairly normal sex lives.

• Bladder problems. Urinary incontinence caused by nerve damage can be difficult to treat. The first step for many people is to change their behavior, urinating more often ("by the clock") to avoid having a full bladder. The goal is to keep the bladder as empty as possible. If this simple measure fails, surgery may be helpful in some cases.

• Low blood pressure (orthostatic hypotension). If you have problems with dizziness or light-headedness when sitting or standing up, you may benefit from behavioral changes. Learning to change positions more slowly, allowing your legs to dangle over the side of the bed for a few minutes before standing up in the morning, and other techniques may be of help. Some people may need to wear high elastic stockings to prevent blood from rushing away from the upper body. Adding salt to your diet may also help raise your blood pressure. The danger of orthostatic hypotension is that it may easily be mistaken for hypoglycemia. Sugar will not alleviate these symptoms and may cause a needless increase in your blood sugar levels.

Large Blood Vessel Disease

There are two main types of diabetic vascular (blood vessel) disease: *microvascular disease* affects the eyes, kidneys, and some nerves, as we've already discussed; *macro- (large) vessel disease* affects the arteries supplying the heart, brain, arms, and legs. Macrovascular disease does not occur only in people with diabetes, but it is much more common in people with IDDM and NIDDM than in people without diabetes. If you have IDDM, your risk of macrovascular disease is high in comparison with people of the same age without diabetes; however, it's still a pretty small risk, unless you have kidney failure. The fact is that very few young people, with or without IDDM, get heart disease or stroke. On the other hand, people with NIDDM, who are generally older, are at risk because of their age, their weight, their high blood pressure, and because they sometimes have cholesterol problems. About one out of four people with NIDDM will have macrovascular complications, which is considerably higher (two to seven times higher) than the rate of macrovascular disease in people without diabetes.

Heart disease causes more than 500,000 deaths each year in the U.S. It is the leading cause of mortality in the United States today, accounting for about half of all deaths, and about one third of all deaths of people between the age of thirty-five and sixty-five. These statistics convey two very important ideas: (1) heart disease is very dangerous, and (2) heart disease is very common.

Heart disease doesn't happen overnight. It's usually a slow, steady process that takes many years before it causes symptoms. Several risk factors for heart disease have been identified in addition to diabetes. One of these is high serum (blood) cholesterol. One reason that people with diabetes have high rates of heart disease is that they frequently have high levels of cholesterol circulating in their bloodstream. That high cholesterol is bad for your health is news to almost no one—studies of large populations in several countries have shown that the higher the level of cholesterol in your blood, the more susceptible you are to heart disease. We've all heard about the "bad" cholesterol (LDL, or *low density lipoprotein*) that causes heart disease and the "good" cholesterol (HDL, or *high density lipoprotein*) that protects against heart disease. People with diabetes, and especially those with NIDDM, tend to have higher levels of the LDL, the bad cholesterol, and lower levels of HDL, the protective cholesterol.

High blood pressure forces your heart to work harder to pump blood through your body, and it has a direct, stressful effect on blood vessel walls. People with diabetes tend to be more susceptible to high blood pressure, which means they're at greater risk for heart disease and stroke.

Smoking is another major risk factor for heart disease and peripheral vascular disease. Diabetes and smoking are, quite literally, a deadly combination.

High cholesterol, high blood pressure, and smoking predispose people to blockages in the vessels supplying the heart, brain, arms, and legs. Although the process isn't completely understood, it appears that the first changes include a buildup of cholesterol and fat in the vessel wall, a condition called *atherosclerosis*. The cholesterol deposit leads to an immune system reaction that results in an inflammatory reaction and more cholesterol-rich cells in the blood vessel wall. Eventually, patches called *plaques* form on the inner surface of the blood vessel, narrowing it and making it harder for blood to pass through. If a clot forms on top of the plaque, it may block off the blood vessel.

Other diabetic complications, particularly kidney disease, also play a role in making heart disease more common among people with diabetes. In addition to the high blood pressure and high cholesterol that accompany kidney failure, the increase in waste products that the damaged kidneys fail to filter out has a direct effect on the formation of plaques. People with kidney failure may have a twenty- to thirtyfold greater risk for heart disease than people without kidney disease.

When blood fails to reach the heart muscle, it's called a *myocardial infarction* (MI), or heart attack. During a heart attack, portions of your heart muscle become starved of blood and oxygen and start to die. A heart attack is probably the most serious manifestation of heart disease, because it usually comes without warning, irreversibly destroys heart muscle, and frequently kills before there's time to do anything about it.

Although peripheral vascular disease does not cause

heart attacks, it is still as serious a complication as any of the others we've talked about. Peripheral vascular disease is similar to the vascular disease of the heart, but it affects the blood vessels supplying the brain, other organs and, in particular, the legs and feet. Most peripheral vascular disease involves clogging and closing of arteries, which leaves vulnerable tissues without an adequate blood supply, explains Dr. Glenn LaMuraglia, a vascular surgeon at Mass General who sees many patients with diabetes and peripheral vascular disease.

"The most common problem we see," he says, "is obstruction of the circulation in their legs, or obstruction of the circulation in the arteries to their brain, the *carotid arteries*. The same obstructions may occur in the intestines, the kidneys, or the arms, although these are less common."

As we've mentioned, peripheral vascular disease can combine with other complications to create even more severe health problems. For instance, the combination of poor circulation, sensory neuropathy in the feet, and poor eyesight makes foot care a challenge and a source of concern for many people with diabetes. Diabetes is the most frequent cause of amputations in the United States; people with diabetes are 20 to 30 times more likely to undergo an amputation than people without diabetes. We'll talk about this more in the following section, Foot Problems and Care.

Although peripheral vascular disease is unlikely to be fatal—except when it causes a stroke—it can cause some other problems that may require hospitalization and perhaps intensive therapy to avoid amputation. The all-too-common results of peripheral vascular disease include the following:

• Symptoms from decreased blood flow. When the requirements for blood flow to the heart muscle, which increase with exercise and increased heart rate, cannot be met because the blood supply to this muscle is blocked, patients often develop chest pain or pressure, called *angina*. Similarly, when exercising leg muscles aren't supplied with enough blood, patients develop a cramping, painful sensation in the muscle called *intermittent claudication*. The calf muscle is most commonly affected, but depending on which arteries are blocked, pain in the thighs or buttocks can occur. Intermittent claudication characteristically affects one leg more than the other. (This is different from sensory neuropathy, in which both sides are affected similarly.) The symptoms occur when you exercise and generally stop after a few minutes of rest. If you have peripheral vascular disease, the amount of time or distance that you'll be able to walk before developing leg pain is usually fairly consistent and can be used as an indicator as to how severe the obstruction of blood flow in your leg is. (If you can walk only shorter distances before you feel leg pain, you have a more severe blockage.) As the vascular blockage worsens, the time and distance that you can walk without pain decreases.

The ultimate manifestation of peripheral vascular disease is pain at rest. If your pain progresses to the point that it still occurs when you are sitting, this means that the blood supply to your muscles is so poor that it persists even when you're not exercising.

• Foot ulcers. As I mentioned previously, most foot ulcers begin because of undetected trauma when you have peripheral neuropathy. Blood flow that has diminished considerably can also lead to, or contribute to, the development and worsening of foot ulcers. The parts of the foot that are farthest "downstream"—the toes—are most commonly affected, but poor circulation can also promote or worsen diabetic foot ulcers in any part of the foot or even above the foot.

Limited circulation will adversely affect the ability of an amputation to heal. If blood flow is not adequate for healing at a certain amputation level, for example, your doctor may attempt to bring greater blood flow to the amputation area (with a bypass procedure, described later in this section) or select a higher amputation site, closer to adequate blood supply.

• Strokes and transient ischemic attacks (TIAs). Like the heart and legs, the brain is dependent on a continuous, reliable supply of oxygen and nutrients. Unlike the two sets of muscles we have already discussed, the blood flow to the brain changes only minimally with its workload (otherwise known as "thinking"). If the blood supply to the brain is decreased or cut for even a brief period, the destruction of brain tissue can wreak devastating effects. The blood vessels that carry blood to the brain are the carotid and the vertebral arteries. Blockage of these vessels or smaller vessels within the brain itself are more common in IDDM and NIDDM, which is why there is increased risk of stroke in these patients.

Different areas of the brain control different functions; the specific type of damage (paralysis, loss of speech, severe dizziness, or sensory changes) depends on which area of the brain is deprived of blood supply. As with angina and heart disease, there are warning signs of stroke and vascular diseases. If blood flow decreases transiently, but not for a long enough time to destroy brain tissue, a *transient ischemic attack* (TIA) may occur. These episodes can last for minutes to hours. People may have similar symptoms from these attacks on several different occasions, such as recurrent left arm weakness. TIAs may occur with the formation of small clots that temporarily block a narrowed vessel, or they may accompany changes in blood pressure. They are a serious warning sign of a serious problem and should be reported immediately to your physician. Unfortunately, hypoglycemia can cause similar transient symptoms. It's very important to check your blood sugar any time you have peculiar symptoms that could be hypoglycemia, to determine whether low blood sugar is the cause, and seek appropriate therapy.

Diagnosis

As we've learned more about causes, prevention, and treatment of heart disease and peripheral vascular disease, early diagnosis has become increasingly important. Heart disease is a highly preventable cause of death, and the earlier you identify it, the easier it is for you and your physician to do something about it.

Although the mechanisms are not always known, we now have a fairly definitive list of the causes of heart disease. We refer to these causes as *risk factors* because in people with these characteristics, heart disease is significantly more likely to appear. The major risk factors are:

- smoking
- high blood pressure
- high LDL cholesterol and low HDL cholesterol
- family history of heart disease
- diabetes
- obesity (being more than 20 percent over your ideal weight range)

Notice that diabetes is, itself, one of the risk factors. If you have any other of these risk factors, the likelihood of your having heart disease has increased dramatically. Remember that people with diabetes, and especially NIDDM, very often have high blood pressure, low HDL cholesterol, high LDL cholesterol, and obesity. Thus they may already be stuck with three or four risk factors. Perhaps we doctors don't say it often enough, but keep in mind that if you're a diabetic and you smoke, you're sending an invitation to heart disease—smoking adds another risk factor and increases the incidence of all forms of macrovascular disease.

Although in the general population heart disease is more common in men than in women, among people with diabetes, men and women have similar risks of developing heart disease. I can't stress enough the seriousness of this disease. If you have any of the following symptoms of heart disease, you should contact your physician and/or go to an emergency room as soon as possible:

- uncomfortable pressure or squeezing in the chest, especially with exercise
- severe chest pain
- pain that spreads to the shoulders, neck, or arms and hands
- light-headedness or irregular heartbeat
- fainting
- sweating or nausea with chest discomfort
- difficulty breathing

To determine whether heart disease has caused your symptoms, and to determine the severity of heart disease and how well your heart is working, your doctor may also ask you to undergo an *electrocardiogram,* often called an EKG. The EKG helps determine whether there is any existing damage to your heart by measuring the heart's electrical patterns. Certain identifiable changes in the heart's electrical signaling take place during *angina* (decreased blood flow to the heart), during an *acute myocardial infarction* (heart attack), and even long after a heart attack. By analyzing your EKG, your physician can determine whether your symptoms are likely to be a result of heart disease. During the EKG, sensors are attached to several points on your chest and to your arms. It is entirely safe and painless and usually requires just a few minutes to perform.

The EKG, while useful, is not as sensitive as some other tests. When patients feel their symptoms only during exercise—when the rapidly beating heart muscle needs more blood—they may need an *exercise tolerance test,* or *stress test,* to determine whether blood vessels are blocked and how severely. This test is usually performed on a treadmill while the EKG is continuously measured. You will be asked to walk at an increasing rate until your symptoms, including fatigue, shortness of breath, and chest discomfort, force you to stop, or until the doctor or technician supervising the test says you can stop. There are variations on this exercise test; sometimes you'll be given a small amount of radioactive material, called *thallium,* which can identify areas of the heart that have scars from old heart attacks. An ultrasound test, a kind of sonar test of the heart in which sound waves are used to make a picture of the heart, can also be performed during exercise. Finally, continuous (or ambulatory) EKG monitoring is also used to detect heart disease.

If heart disease is suspected on the basis of your medical

history and the results of these tests, additional studies that are more invasive may be needed. All of the tests I've described so far are normally performed without inserting tubes into your veins. A *cardiac catheterization* involves putting a long catheter through an artery and threading it through large blood vessels until it reaches the arteries that supply your heart muscle with blood. A chemical that is easily seen on an x-ray, called a *contrast dye,* is then injected into these arteries so that your doctor, with the help of a *cardiologist,* can see which vessels are narrowed or blocked and to what extent. This information helps determine whether you need surgery, a *coronary artery bypass graft* (CABG), to bring more blood to the parts of the heart that are poorly supplied.

All of the tests above are performed frequently in people with diabetes for two reasons. First, diabetes makes heart disease more likely, and since it is potentially fatal, your physician will aggressively try to detect it. Second, people with diabetes, especially if they have neuropathy, may have few or no warning symptoms of heart disease, even when it is present. Therefore, doctors tend to use these diagnostic tests liberally with their diabetes patients.

Peripheral vascular disease is often diagnosed from your medical history and physical examination. Your doctor will often feel for pulses in your neck, ankles, and feet. This provides a rough guide as to whether there is blockage in the arteries and whether adequate quantities of blood are reaching your feet. In addition, other changes occur if your blood supply is severely limited. For example, if your feet turn very red when you sit up with your legs hanging down, or if they are blue and cold, you may have a severe obstruction in the blood flow to your legs and feet. Don't try to diagnose or treat these problems yourself; your doctor should examine your feet on a regular basis for these changes. There are also tests that can measure altered blood flow to the feet and brain. Comparison of the blood pressure in the ankle to that of the arm provides an index of circulation to the feet. Ultrasound study of the carotid vessels can reveal whether significant blockage exists. When necessary, tests similar to cardiac catheterization can directly check for the presence of blockages in your arteries. Future advances in *magnetic resonance imaging* (MRI) may someday eliminate the need for using these invasive catheters.

Your doctor can determine whether you're at especially high risk for macrovascular disease by testing your blood pressure and your cholesterol. Remember that having diabetes is a risk factor by itself. In addition, being overweight and having a parent or sibling who was found to have heart disease at an early age are considered risk factors. Finally, smoking is an obvious risk factor that doesn't require any diagnostic test to detect.

Treatment

Because heart disease is both common and potentially fatal, causing more deaths than any other disease, there are constant discussions among doctors over the best way to prevent and treat it.

Happily, there have been major advances in the treatment of risk factors that lead to heart disease. A wealth of information suggests that efforts to reduce these risk factors decrease the occurrence or progression of cardiac disease. Unfortunately, many people with diabetes, and almost all people with NIDDM, have multiple risk factors and may need to be treated for obesity, high blood pressure, and abnormal cholesterol levels, not to mention diabetes. Sadly, most of the studies focusing on heart disease prevention have *excluded* people with diabetes. So even though we think that lowering cholesterol and blood pressure is effective in decreasing the development of heart disease, the studies that show this have not adequately addressed the diabetic population. Despite these gaps in information, most physicians have worked hard to help their patients with diabetes lower their blood pressure and cholesterol, lose weight, and get their blood sugar under control.

Although there are many controversies over how to prevent heart disease in people with diabetes, one area in which there is some agreement is the dietary approach. In general, a sensible, low-fat, low-cholesterol diet is preferred (see Dietary Guidelines box for suggested goals). Diet is even more important for people who have elevated total cholesterol or elevated LDL cholesterol. Specific guidelines have been developed to treat these risk factors.

Similarly, a low-salt diet may be the first step in controlling high blood pressure. Finally, exercise can help with weight control and high blood pressure. If your health permits, and under the supervision of your doctor, you might start with about fifteen minutes of low-intensity, low-impact exercise. People with diabetes who also have neuropathy or retinopathy will need to give special consideration to the type of exercise that's best for them (see Chapter 6). Foot care is especially important and, of course, any changes in exercise or diet may have an impact on blood sugar levels. If you smoke, you should try to quit as soon as possible. If you want to prevent heart disease, refer to Chapter 4 on diet and Chapter 6 on exercise and take another look at the guidelines given there. The

Dietary Guidelines to Prevent Heart Disease

For All Diabetic Patients

- Reduce total fat to less than 30 percent of total calories
- Reduce saturated fat to less than 10 percent of total calories
- Reduce cholesterol intake to less than 300 mg per day

For Overweight Type II Diabetes

- Adopt a hypocaloric (reduced calorie) diet to achieve weight loss and blood sugar control—will also improve triglyceride levels

For Hypertensive Diabetic Patients

- Reduce sodium intake to less than 2.5 grams per day

For Diabetic Patients with Abnormal Lipids (cholesterol, triglycerides)

- Reduce saturated fat to less than 7 percent of total calories
- Reduce dietary cholesterol to less than 200 mg per day

American Heart Association offers many cookbooks and guides that address heart disease.

Should diet, exercise, and other simple measures fail to keep your blood pressure and cholesterol in a healthy range, there are a wide variety of drugs that can help bring these risk factors into an acceptable range. Your doctor will usually recommend drug therapy if your LDL choles-

LDL Cholesterol Levels Requiring Therapy in Diabetes			
	DESIRABLE	REQUIRES DIET	REQUIRES DIET & MEDICATION
Diabetes only	<130	>160	>190
1 or more risk factors*	<130	>130	>160
Heart disease	<100	>100	>130

*Risk factors, in addition to diabetes, include male sex, hypertension, smoking, low HDL cholesterol (<35), and family history of premature heart disease. Adapted from National Cholesterol Education Program (NCEP) guidelines.

terol exceeds specific levels, which are based on the number of risk factors you have and whether you have a history of heart disease (see Box above). You may be referred to a cardiologist who will supervise your treatment. Cholesterol-lowering drugs that your doctor may prescribe include:

• Bile acid sequestrants. Used since 1965 to control elevated blood cholesterol, cholestyramine and colestipol are the two most commonly used in this category of drugs that bind cholesterol in the intestine. Normally administered as powders mixed with water or juice, bile acid sequestrants can also be eaten as "candy" bars. Yearly costs average approximately $1,000 for 16 grams of Questran per day or 20 grams of Colestid. The major problems with these safe and effective agents are that they have a consistency like sand and are unpleasant to take. They also commonly cause constipation, which can be bothersome.

• Niacin (nicotinic acid). Niacin is a B vitamin that was discovered in 1955 to have cholesterol-lowering qualities.

It also elevates "good" cholesterol (HDL) levels. Treatment typically begins with 100 to 250 mg/day in a single dose taken after dinner, and the dosage is increased to up to 6 g/day taken in multiple doses. Annual cost of niacin therapy can be as low as $50. However, niacin treatment may worsen glucose control. In addition, many patients have trouble, especially at higher doses, with flushing, itching, and, occasionally, inflammation of the liver. Don't take niacin except under your doctor's supervision.

• HMG-CoA reductase inhibitors. The cost for a year's treatment with an average dose of one of the relatively new HMG-CoA reductase inhibitors is $900. These drugs are the most effective in lowering cholesterol, typically lowering LDL cholesterol by 25 to 30 percent. Patients with hyperlipidemia (an abnormally high amount of lipids [fats] in the blood) and diabetes can use these drugs with relative safety. Lovastatin can be combined with niacin and/or bile acid sequestrants to greater effect. LDL reductions of up to 50 percent have been seen in patients treated with colestipol and lovastatin. As with the bile acid binding agents and niacin before them, HMG-CoA reductase inhibitors have been demonstrated to decrease not only cholesterol levels, but also the incidence of heart disease.

One of the most common abnormal lipid patterns in diabetes is an elevated *triglyceride* level accompanied by a low HDL-cholesterol level. Triglycerides are another form of blood lipid that, like LDL-cholesterol, raise your risk of heart disease. Although there is relatively little one can do to raise HDL (exercise, moderate alcohol intake, and niacin can raise levels slightly), triglyceride levels can be effectively lowered with better control of diabetes and weight loss. Therefore, lowering blood sugar levels should be your first step in lowering triglyceride levels. If dietary and blood sugar lowering efforts don't reduce your triglyceride levels to less than 400 mg/dl, your doctor may prescribe a medication.

• Fibric acids. At the cost of $1,000 for a year's treatment with gemfibrozil, fibric acids effectively lower triglyceride levels in patients with diabetes. A small percentage of patients treated with fibric acids suffer from abdominal pain, diarrhea, and nausea, but these medications are usually well tolerated. Fibric acids do not exacerbate diabetes, and they are necessary for treatment of very high triglyceride levels that may cause pancreatitis.

If you have high blood pressure (hypertension), and a low-salt diet and exercise have failed to lower it, your doctor may decide to use drugs. Some of the more commonly used drugs include:

• Diuretics. Relatively safe and inexpensive, diuretics reduce blood pressure by removing salt from your circulation through the kidneys. In most adults, these drugs are the first line of defense against hypertension. Unfortunately, these drugs may worsen glucose control in people with diabetes and therefore are often avoided.

• ACE inhibitors. Angiotensin-converting enzyme (ACE) inhibitors have been used for more than a decade. They block the formation of a substance that constricts blood vessels and raises blood pressure. These drugs can bring blood pressure into a normal range and can be particularly effective in slowing the progress of kidney disease (see the earlier section in this chapter). ACE inhibitors are considerably more expensive than diuretics. Although usually well tolerated, they can cause headache, dizziness, and cough. ACE inhibitors also may increase potassium levels, so monitoring may be needed, and some people experience a decline in kidney function when the drug is used.

• Calcium channel blockers. These drugs dilate blood vessels to lower blood pressure and allow the heart to beat more easily. Side effects include headache, ankle swelling, dizziness, flushing, and constipation. They are also a relatively expensive, but often necessary, alternative to diuretics. The don't interfere with diabetes control.

There are many other types of drugs used to treat high blood pressure. One group of drugs, the beta-adrenergic blockers, which block the effects of adrenaline and similar substances, are effective at treating both high blood pressure and heart disease. Unfortunately, they have several side effects that are particularly troublesome for people with diabetes. Beta-blockers decrease insulin secretion and can worsen blood sugar control in people with NIDDM. In addition, they can prolong recovery from hypoglycemia. Therefore, you should take special care if you're taking insulin or sulfo-nylureas and your doctor prescribes beta blockers. Although physicians often try to avoid using them to treat high blood pressure in patients with diabetes, sometimes they are prescribed for people with both diabetes and heart disease.

Surgical Intervention

As I pointed out earlier, when heart disease has progressed to the point at which major blood vessels supplying the heart muscle (the *coronary arteries*) are critically blocked, surgery may be suggested as an option to bring more blood to the heart and to improve heart function. Probably the most widely used procedure to treat coronary artery disease is the *coronary artery bypass graft* (CABG, or "cabbage" as it's often called). In this procedure, diseased, clogged sections of blood vessels are bypassed with vessels that are moved, or grafted, from other parts of the body, usually the leg or chest wall. The new vessels bring a new supply of blood to specific areas of the heart. Frequently, three or more vessels will be replaced. The new vessels may function for a few years or for many years, depending on various factors. Patients are often treated with aspirin or other anti-clotting drugs to help preserve the function of these new blood vessels. In addition, elevated cholesterol, blood pressure, and other factors that may have led to the blockage of the original, diseased vessel are treated aggressively to prevent the same process from occurring in the new vessel.

Another procedure that has been used with increasing frequency is *angioplasty*. During catheterization, selected vessels that are only partially damaged are expanded by inserting a small collapsed balloon through the obstructed section. The balloon is then inflated until the thickened area is "squashed" alongside the wall. Although this nonsurgical approach is often effective, the dilated area may become blocked within a relatively brief time (hours to months), requiring a repeat balloon procedure or a CABG. Recent studies have suggested that patients with diabetes have better outcomes with a CABG than angio-plasty. After heart surgery, a period of rehabilitation that includes dietary instruction and supervised exercise is important.

Peripheral vascular disease prevention starts with a healthy diet and abstention from tobacco. If clotting is considered a threat to your health, your doctor may suggest that you regularly take aspirin, or another blood thinner such as Coumadin, to reduce your blood's clotting ability. Exercise up to the point where pain begins is encouraged with the hope that *collateral circulation* (circulation through other, smaller blood vessels) will develop, bringing more blood to the muscles.

If your peripheral vascular disease becomes severe, there are surgical treatments in some cases that may improve your ability to exercise or may reduce the risk of stroke and carotid disease. For instance, if the carotid arteries that supply the brain with blood become clogged, your doctor may suggest that you undergo a *carotid endarterectomy*. In this procedure, these blood vessels are opened up and cleaned out. We'll talk more about treatments for peripheral vascular disease of the feet and lower legs in the next section.

Foot Problems and Care

We've already learned a little bit about how complications tend to combine to exacerbate one another. For example, kidney disease raises the risk of heart disease. Similarly, the feet and lower legs are affected by neuropathy and vascular disease. The unfortunate result is that diabetes causes more amputations than any other disease. As a person with diabetes, you need to make sure that every regular visit to your doctor includes a close examination of your feet, and *you* must be conscious of your feet and the potential for injury to them every day.

Let's think for a minute about how you normally protect your feet from injuries and infections. Let's say you're walking on the beach in bare feet and step on a piece of glass. First, you feel the pain of getting cut. You stop walking and bend over to take a look at your foot. There's blood seeping out, and you're worried about infection, so you rinse it out with salt water and find something clean to put on it. Then you walk back, being careful to avoid putting your full weight on the injured foot. Soon, you'll have a doctor look at the foot and with time and care, your foot will be back to normal.

If you have diabetes, the picture can be completely different. That's because the complications of diabetes have ways of blunting each one of these defense mechanisms. Here's how:

Once again, you're barefoot on the beach and cut your foot. If you're a person with diabetic neuropathy, you might not feel the cut at first, in which case you would continue to walk for a while on your cut foot. While you do, sand and grime get into the cut. You may realize that you have an injury only when you notice blood on your sock, or only when your entire foot becomes swollen. If you have diabetic retinopathy, your vision of the cut may not be clear. If you have peripheral vascular disease and the circulation to your foot is poor, any infection or ulcer is likely to become more severe. Poor blood supply means that the foot tissue is starved for nutrients. Also, immune cells and antibiotics that fight infection may not reach the affected areas. The infection invades deeper into the foot, blood supply grows worse, and the risk of amputation becomes greater.

That's the worst-case scenario. It's not intended to frighten you but to demonstrate how these complications of diabetes—vascular disease, neuropathy, and retinopathy—all contribute to make foot care difficult.

That's why you need to take special care of your feet, particularly if you have diabetic neuropathy, vascular disease, or any other condition that might make it difficult for you to detect problems or changes in your feet. Dr. Robert Scardina is chief of podiatry at Mass General, and he specializes in the care and prevention of foot problems. We talked with him about the problems that people with diabetes sometimes have in taking care of their feet.

"It's not uncommon for a person with neuropathy to feel as if he is *physically separated* from an extremity," he says. "People with neuropathy often have numbness in their feet, what we call *insensitive feet*. The lack of sensation means that at the nervous system level—and sometimes at the psychological level—there's actually a disconnection between the person and foot. We try to emphasize to patients that they've lost one sensory component or one way of identifying problems with their feet. Now they have to compensate.

"How do you compensate? With your own eyes, with a mirror, with the help of a family member. Since you've lost the red flag of pain (the most important way of recognizing foot problems), you've got to learn to compensate with some others."

The first thing you need to do is to start spending more time looking at and caring for your feet. One way to do this is to wash your feet every day. "Don't soak them," Dr. Scardina says. "Soaking will dry your skin out and leave it vulnerable to cracking. Wash them in warm, soapy water that is not too hot. Test the temperature of the water with your finger or wrist. When you're done wash-

ing your feet, dry them well with a towel, including between the toes."

Now, in a well-lit space, inspect your feet. You're looking for small cuts, bruises, corns, unexplained bumps,
sores, calluses; anything that looks at all out of the ordinary. Perhaps you can't see the bottom of your feet without bending over.

"When I talk to patients, I emphasize the need for attention to the foot, and that a friend or family member
and certain devices can help you give the foot attention,"
Dr. Scardina says. "Injuries at both ends of the temperature spectrum are not uncommon: feet can be damaged by
both cold and heat. I just saw a patient who injured himself by sleeping with his foot right next to a heater. These
are things that you have to try to foresee and prevent. For
instance, if you can't trust your own sense of temperature
to tell you when your bathwater is too hot, use a ther-
mometer."

Another thing you should try to prevent, or take care of
should it arise, is *dry skin* on your feet. Undermoisturized
skin is vulnerable to cracking and even bleeding. Depending on heredity, your shoes, the kind of socks you wear,
and the kind of work you do, you might need to moistur-
ize your feet several times a day to avoid injury. There are
a number of over-the-counter creams you can use to keep
the skin on your feet moist and healthy, such as Nivea and
Alpha-Keri. Some of my patients with very dry skin prefer
Eucerin because it's very thick and doesn't rub off easily.

"Pay close attention to your heels, because this is a spot
where dryness and cracking can lead to some very serious
injuries," Dr. Scardina says. "If your heels are very dry,
rub them with cream before going to bed and then cover
them with plastic wrap to hold the moisture in. Try leav-

ing them that way overnight for a few nights, until they become moister."

Another way to give your feet some preventive attention is in your footwear selection. Wear comfortable shoes, avoiding high heels or any shoe that pinches your toes or heels. Wear socks whenever possible, or stockings at the very least, but don't walk around in bare feet, or with bare feet inside of shoes. (This is true even on the beach, as illustrated by our previous example.) If your feet become insensitive, you may want to try wearing shoes with extra cushioning, like running or walking shoes. Some people change their shoes once a day, just to change the stress patterns on their feet and to give themselves an opportunity to inspect their feet for injuries. For people with very bad feet, there is the "space shoe," a customized shoe that gives more space for different kinds of deformities.

"Don't buy tight shoes thinking that you can break them in," Dr. Scardina says. "While the shoes are stretching, your foot is being mashed against the sides of the shoe. Take home shoes that fit comfortably the day you buy them."

If you have diabetes, ordinary things like taking care of your toenails become more important to the health of your feet and to your overall health. A poorly manicured toenail can be a "foothold" where fungus and other types of infections get started. A sharp-edged nail that presses against the adjacent toe is a common cause of toe ulcers. If you can't reach your toenails or can't see them well, recruit a friend or family member to help you. Your physician may recommend a podiatrist.

The same goes for calluses and corns. Skin that becomes thickened by unusual stress patterns can lead to infections. You may need to seek a podiatrist's help for treatment. In some cases, pads can help prevent calluses and corns. Again, you may need someone to help you keep an eye on these injuries, and on cuts and scratches, too. Don't perform surgery on your own feet!

It can sound a little ridiculous, or even self-indulgent, asking someone you know to cut your toenails for you. But keep in mind that it's for your own good health, and it could save you a lot of trouble in the long run. If you think that it's a lot of trouble to find someone to cut your toenails, think how much worse it could be if your foot were infected, and you needed surgery to take care of it. It could mean weeks on crutches, or even in a wheelchair. This is the kind of trade-off you have to make, and why you have to be so patient and careful with diabetes.

Another foot problem that people with diabetes need to be alert to is *Charcot foot* (also sometimes known as *Charcot neuroarthropathy*). This general breakdown in the skeletal architecture of the foot occurs quite insidiously, after even a slight foot injury. People who already suffer from severe peripheral diabetic neuropathy are most vulnerable. If you injure your foot or have unexplained swelling, you should be seen by your doctor immediately. If Charcot foot is diagnosed, you may have to keep weight off the foot for up to sixteen weeks; bed rest and special footwear may be recommended.

"When someone has some of the five Ps, then it's time to get more aggressive," Dr. Scardina says. "The five Ps are pain, pallor (paleness), paresthesia (abnormal feeling such as numbness), no pulses, and paralysis. When we see someone with several or all of these five Ps, we may send that person to a vascular surgeon for evaluation and treatment."

With proper foot care, you can do much to decrease the risk of complications and perhaps live your entire life without serious diabetic foot problems. Remember, the first step in all of this is tight blood sugar control, because that's how the complications that lead to foot problems—neuropathy, vascular disease, and retinopathy—get started in the first place. Try to be patient, more patient even than diabetes is, and live a complication-free life.

9

Diabetes and Pregnancy

It was a warm day in September and I was speaking with one of my patients, a young woman I've known for many years who was diagnosed with insulin-dependent diabetes (type I or IDDM) in her late twenties. Joan had grown up in a small town in a farming region of Connecticut. Although she'd lived in Boston for several years, she still carried with her the sincerity and openness that reflected the quiet, open spaces of her upbringing.

As an experienced nurse at one of Boston's teaching hospitals, Joan had seen the ravages of diabetes and knew full well the complications that could occur. She was also aware that diabetes self-care was a tough, time-consuming practice, and that even the very best self-care couldn't always protect her completely from hypoglycemia, or from the long-term complications of diabetes. Despite having learned that she was suffering from a chronic disease that would demand constant care for the rest of her life, Joan was less disturbed by the medical issues than by the emotional ones. Already a modest, self-effacing person by nature, the diagnosis led to a period of self-criticism. She began to make some assumptions about herself and her future that, in retrospect, were false and destructive.

"I began to feel that I was damaged goods, that I was not as good as I once was," Joan told me. "I thought that no one would ever want to be close to me, to share my life with diabetes, because I was at risk for all these horrible complications. I felt excluded from all kinds of things. I think the hardest thing for me to face was the idea of having children. I was convinced that I would never have children, either because I would never get married, or because the complications of diabetes would be too severe."

Many people with diabetes have expressed similar fears to me. They worry about the strain that pregnancy might put on their kidneys, and whether pregnancy will cause permanent kidney damage or worsen their eyesight. They worry that their child might not be healthy at birth or may develop diabetes later in life. Women with diabetes often need reassurance that they're eligible for a chance to have a healthy, happy, normal baby.

There once was a time when no one, patient or physician, was confident about the outcome of pregnancy in women with diabetes. Years ago, many doctors urged their female patients with diabetes not to attempt pregnancy. The fear of pregnancy was such that sterilization was sometimes suggested as a safety measure.

There are some instances, relatively rare, when pregnancy may add a lot of risk for maternal well-being. For instance, a woman who has had a kidney transplant and is already suffering from high blood pressure and severe eye disease might be at too high a risk for a successful pregnancy. Acquiring and maintaining a transplanted kidney is a long, tough process. Many people who have gone to the trouble to get a new kidney might not want to risk losing it in a complicated pregnancy. Some people with diabetic retinopathy may not want to risk further damage to their eyes.

Gail Denman, the patient at Mass General's Diabetes Center who was introduced in Chapter 2, decided several years ago that she would not try to become pregnant. "It's a little frustrating because it's beyond my control," she told me. Gail has had several operations to try to restore some of her eyesight, much of which has been lost to diabetic retinopathy. "I'm over the hard part now. Stabilizing my complications was hard. It was difficult. I was taking care of myself as best I could. But the risk to my health from pregnancy was just too great."

Decisions about pregnancy are extremely private and individual, and they should be made in consultation with qualified specialists in diabetes, obstetrics, and, if necessary, kidney or eye treatment. However, with current methods of monitoring and self-treatment, most women with diabetes who are willing to put in the necessary time and effort to keep their blood sugars in the recommended range before and during pregnancy have almost the same chance of delivering a healthy baby as women without diabetes. The risk to the mother is usually small, unless advanced kidney or eye disease is present. Although diabetic eye damage and the amount of protein that leaks into the urine may worsen during pregnancy, they can usually be managed fairly easily. Most of the adverse changes that develop during pregnancy reverse after delivery and have no long-term impact.

There are several types of diabetes that affect pregnancy.

Insulin-dependent diabetic women who decide to become pregnant must make special efforts to prepare for their pregnancy and control their blood sugar in a very tight range before and during pregnancy. Clinical research has demonstrated that diabetic women who achieve this goal do very well during pregnancy and have an excellent chance of having a healthy baby. Relatively few women with non-insulin-dependent diabetes (NIDDM) are in their childbearing years, because NIDDM usually develops during the later years of life. However, women who belong to certain minority groups, such as Mexican Americans or American Indians, in which NIDDM is especially common may develop NIDDM while still fertile. A woman with NIDDM who becomes pregnant must aim for the same tight control as pregnant women with IDDM. Specialized diets and insulin therapy are usually recommended.

A third type of diabetes occurs *only* during pregnancy, and it usually resolves after delivery. Gestational diabetes (GDM) occurs in 3 to 5 percent of all pregnancies, usually beginning in the late second or early third trimester (i.e., after week 24). Women are now routinely tested between weeks 24 and 28 of pregnancy with a standard screening glucose tolerance test (see page 223 later in this chapter). Those who test positive on the screening test have a more definitive test performed. If you are diagnosed with GDM, proper diet is often the only treatment necessary. You may need insulin for the final two or three months of your pregnancy. GDM usually disappears almost immediately after delivery. However, women who have had GDM are at high risk to develop NIDDM later in life and should be monitored on a regular basis.

Taking Care of Your Diabetes While You Are Pregnant

You've probably guessed by now that the first thing that I'll mention is the importance of tight blood sugar control. It's no exaggeration to say that this is probably one of the most important facets of your self-care during pregnancy. If you have IDDM or NIDDM and know you want to become pregnant, you should seek out the care of a diabetes treatment team so that you can begin getting your blood sugar under the best control possible *before* you become

---

Guidelines for Diabetes Care During Pregnancy

For Women with Diabetes Before Pregnancy

- Plan your pregnancies.
- Optimize blood glucose control before pregnancy and maintain tight glucose goals during early pregnancy to decrease malformations in newborn.
- Maintain tight glucose control for rest of pregnancy to decrease "large-for-date" babies and other complications at the time of delivery.
- Diet and insulin must be adjusted to account for increased caloric requirements as baby grows. Insulin requirements increase dramatically in the last half of pregnancy and then decrease during labor and after delivery.
- Maintain tight control after delivery for your health. Adjust your diet to account for the increased calories required for breast feeding.
- Eye and kidney status should be carefully followed during pregnancy, especially if you had complications before pregnancy.

For Women Who Develop Diabetes During Pregnancy (Gestational Diabetes)

- If you are overweight, consult with your physician regarding desirable weight gain for pregnancy.
- Follow diet therapy and sugar-monitoring schedule.
- If blood sugar levels are not in a desirable range (before and after meals), you may need insulin. Usually given as one or two daily injections with a combination of intermediate- and rapid-acting insulins.

AFTER DELIVERY
- Oral glucose tolerance test should be performed approximately two months after delivery.
- Blood sugar should be measured regularly (annually).
- Decrease risk for future development of diabetes by achieving and maintaining ideal body weight.

For All Pregnant Women

- Screening (50 gram) oral glucose tolerance test between week 24 and 28 of pregnancy.
- Definitive (100 gram) oral glucose tolerance test for women with one hour glucose result $\geq$ 140 mg/dl on screening test.

pregnant. For women with diabetes, unfortunately, unplanned pregnancies are much riskier.

Tight blood sugar control is *essential* for the health of your fetus. In the past, one of the main differences between pregnancies in women with and in those without diabetes was the rate of fetal death and abnormalities. The higher the levels of blood sugar, the higher the rates of miscarriage and of birth defects—often called *congenital malformations*. These malformations can include both minor and major birth defects, from webbed toes, to a malformed kidney, or to something as serious as incomplete formation of the central nervous system, called *neural tube defects.*

Drs. Michael Greene and Bob Blatman are two of the obstetricians at Mass General who specialize in "high-risk" obstetrics. At Mass General, all pregnant women with diabetes are classified as high-risk. This may sound scary, but it is a precaution designed to give them special attention. Dr. Blatman summarizes the importance of tight blood sugar control before and during pregnancy:

"The rate of congenital malformations in the general population is about 2 to 2.5 percent," he says. "When we divide our patients into low, medium, and high sugar groups—the low being in the best blood sugar control, and the high in the poorest control—the patients in the low group have the least risk of congenital malformations. It's about 3 percent, only a little higher than the rate in mothers without diabetes. Mothers in the medium group do pretty well, too. Their rate of congenital malformations is a little higher, in the 4 percent range.

"However, patients in the high group have a much higher rate. About 15 to 20 percent of pregnancies in patients who have poor blood sugar control have children with congenital malformations. The important thing to remember is that the better you take care of your blood sugar, the better you take care of your baby."

Keep in mind that the fetus takes some of its most important developmental steps during the first six weeks of pregnancy, when most of the major organs are formed. At this stage, many of the body's main features are sketched out. The eyes and spine are already recognizable at the end of these first six weeks. (For a close look at the developing fetus through a photographer's eye, see *A Child Is Born,* by Lennart Nilsson.)

Since most women don't even know they are pregnant until week three of conception—one week after their period normally would have started—it is important that they have good glucose control *before* they decide to become pregnant. Some women go a couple of months without knowing that they're carrying a child. Being in tight blood glucose control *before* pregnancy begins ensures that your baby will have the benefit of a healthy environment from the very first day of conception.

Remember that even if, for whatever reason, you find out that a couple of weeks of your pregnancy have passed without tight blood sugar control, it's never too late to start working on getting your blood sugar down into a safe range. If you find that you're pregnant and you've been in poor control, get yourself into the care of a diabetes specialist as soon as you possibly can. By doing this, you can help diminish your baby's risk of congenital malformations. The glycohemoglobin test can help assess your fetus's risk for birth defects. When your doctor determines the level early in pregnancy, he or she can tell you whether your baby is at high risk or not. If the baby *is* at high risk, you can decide whether or not to continue the pregnancy.

If you have been pregnant before and have had a problem with neural tube defects in the fetus, your doctor may recommend that you take *folate,* a vitamin B derivative, *before* you become pregnant. Folate has been shown to reduce the risk of neural tube defects. You should begin taking it before you conceive to ensure that the fetus will receive the benefit of this vitamin from the earliest days of its development.

For most women with diabetes, pregnancy is a wonderful time of life, just as it would be for anyone. Pregnancy is a time when you can become aware of and in touch with your own body, as well as with the fetus developing inside. Naturally, it demands planning and hard work, hopefully after at least a little pleasure, but again, this is true for all women, whether they have diabetes or not.

The first thing I urge pregnant women with diabetes to do is to get into the care of a multidisciplinary pregnancy team. This team would include an obstetrician, like Dr. Greene or Dr. Blatman, a diabetologist (see Chapter 3), a diabetic nurse educator, and a nutritionist. At certain times during your pregnancy, you may need to see other specialists, such as radiologists, who administer the frequent ultrasounds that are the rule to check on the development of the fetus in diabetic women.

Discovering that you are pregnant can happen in all kinds of ways. Hopefully, you will have prepared by keeping your blood sugar control at its best. You may find out you're pregnant during a routine doctor's appointment. You may notice changes that signal pregnancy: a missed period, morning sickness, fatigue, and change in appetite may tip you off. Or, if you're trying to get pregnant, there are a number of home pregnancy tests, many of which are fairly reliable if used correctly. Even after you've used one of these home tests, your doctor may want to corroborate it with a quick laboratory test.

Once it's been established that you're pregnant, congratulations! At Mass General, we usually schedule an introductory visit during which you meet all the members of the team—diabetologist, dietitian, obstetrician, nurse educator, and others—so that you can start to feel comfortable with everyone on the team, and find out a little bit about how we're going to proceed. We'll also determine your due date, which we'll do by finding out the first day of your last period and adding forty weeks to that date. Although this probably won't be the exact date that the baby will arrive, we can use it to approximate when the fetus should hit certain developmental milestones.

In all high-risk pregnancies, which would include any involving diabetes, we usually schedule an early ultrasound. This noninvasive, painless imaging test helps us determine the baby's development, and it can be used to look for congenital malformations.

It's not unusual for clinics specializing in diabetes treatment to admit patients to the hospital early to maximize their diabetes care and implement intensive therapy if they are not already on it. A typical hospital admission to intensify your diabetes control would require two to five days. Depending on your success in achieving tight control, you may need to be admitted more than once. Weekly and monthly visits and frequent telephone contact allow your diabetologist to closely monitor your sugars. Many effective treatment teams include a nurse educator and a nutritionist who will help you adjust your therapy and understand the relationship among food, exercise, and insulin requirements. If you have NIDDM during pregnancy, you will almost certainly need insulin. But as with treatment in the nonpregnant state, the insulin therapy required to achieve normal glucose levels will be less intensive than in IDDM. Many pregnant women with diabetes have persistent problems with low blood sugar (hypoglycemia), and your treatment team can also help you limit their occurrence and treat them (see Hypoglycemia, Chapter 7).

Episodes of hypoglycemia during the first trimester

(three months) of pregnancy are especially common, probably because your body is getting acclimated to intensive therapy. (In light of the DCCT, most women should be aiming for tight control all the time, so hopefully preparing for pregnancy shouldn't mean a major change in your diabetes care.) As your pregnancy progresses, your placenta will begin to make hormones that counteract the effects of insulin. Typically, your insulin requirements increase by one-and-one-half- to two-fold during the final two months of pregnancy. This is an expected normal change.

Although hypoglycemia may be less common during the latter part of pregnancy, it is always a potential danger. As I've said before, there is no way to prevent hypoglycemia completely, so it's best to be prepared for it. Talk with your spouse, friends, and coworkers frankly and explicitly about how to recognize and cope with severe hypoglycemia. *Make sure you have a supply of readily available carbohydrate. You should also have glucagon available, and make sure that people around you know how to use it.* Post emergency numbers near the telephone. Include your own phone number and address on that list, just in case they're hard to remember in a crisis. Keep juice in the refrigerator and hard candies near the bed, in your car, and at your desk. Monitor your blood sugar frequently—remember, symptoms are often misleading. The surest way to know your blood sugar is to test it with your monitor.

Some patients do better on the pump than with multiple injections. Carmella Clark, whom you met in Chapter 2, went on the pump in order to control her blood sugar during pregnancy, and she was extremely happy with her experience.

"My self-care has improved a great deal since I went on the pump," she told me. "I learned so much more about what you should and should not do to keep blood sugars in line, and what levels are healthy for the baby. After my daughter was born, I went back to injecting insulin four times a day. But when I get pregnant again, I'd like to go back on the pump."

As your pregnancy progresses beyond the early stages, your doctors will be paying attention to many important aspects of fetal development. Two in particular that they have to keep a watch on are the fetus's weight and the maturity of its lungs. Fetuses of mothers with diabetes in poor glucose control tend to grow very large in the womb. Even when the mother's blood sugar is under relatively *good* control, birth weights of 10, 11, and 12 pounds are not uncommon. Dr. Blatman told me that the largest baby he had delivered from a mother with diabetes was 12 pounds, 9 ounces. And the baby weighed this a week and a half before its due date!

Size can be a concern. Large babies are harder to deliver than small babies because it's harder to fit them through the birth canal. When babies get especially large—in the 9-pound and above range—it gets more and more difficult to get their shoulders out of the womb. Sometimes, the baby's shoulder gets stuck behind the mother's pubic bone, a situation known as *shoulder dystocia*. The baby will be unable to progress down the birth canal any farther until the dystocia is taken care of.

The most reliable way to minimize the chance of a difficult delivery and possible shoulder dystocia is to induce the mother to deliver the baby a couple of weeks before the due date—before the baby becomes too large. A lot of the baby's growth occurs during the last three or four weeks of pregnancy. If the baby is delivered one or two weeks early, there's usually not too much difference in the baby's overall health, and the chance of a shoulder dystocia or other complications can be drastically reduced.

This is in fact what frequently happens in diabetic pregnancy. A week or two before the due date, if the baby's lungs are mature (see later in this section how this is determined), your obstetrician may call you into the labor and delivery ward and administer a drug called *pitocin*, which sets the mechanisms of labor in motion. Within a matter of hours, contractions begin and the induced delivery takes place. It's similar to the events at the end of any normal pregnancy, except they occur a little earlier, making delivery safer for you and your baby.

However, delivering babies early carries some risk as well. The maturation of the lungs, which allows them to inflate and stay expanded, takes place very late in pregnancy. Babies who are born before their lungs are capable of functioning outside the womb can develop severe health problems. They can't absorb the oxygen they need, and their lungs are particularly vulnerable to infection. If their lungs are very immature, they often need to spend at least a couple of days in the neonatal intensive care unit (NICU), and sometimes weeks or months of such care are necessary.

Thus, there are two competing interests that the obstetrician has to take into account when thinking about how soon to deliver your baby: avoiding problems associated with delivering a larger baby, and avoiding problems associated with immature lungs.

"The simplest way to look at it is that we're trying to avoid birth trauma of any kind," Dr. Blatman says.

"There are no hard-and-fast rules about predicting whether a baby will have birth trauma. There are some small babies who have shoulder dystocias, and some large babies who come shooting right out. There are larger babies who have immature lungs and smaller babies whose lungs are all ready to go."

One tool that's commonly used to predict the fetus's stage of development is ultrasound. This is a relatively new technology that uses sound waves to form a "sonar" picture of the developing fetus. Most pregnant women with diabetes have several ultrasound imaging sessions before they deliver. As I said, ultrasound is completely painless, poses no known risk to you or the fetus, and can actually be fun. It's delightful to see your little fetus moving around, its heart beating and legs kicking, while the various parts of its body slowly take shape and mature. You may be able to determine its sex if your baby is in the right position. Most ultrasound machines can even make prenatal "baby pictures" for you to take home.

From the ultrasound image, your radiologist may be able to make early determinations about whether your fetus is suffering from a congenital abnormality. Another way of testing for such abnormalities is with a test called *amniocentesis*. This is a relatively well-established test that involves taking very small amounts of amniotic fluid from the womb so that genetic analysis can be performed. In addition, toward the end of pregnancy, chemical analysis of the amniotic fluid provides an accurate index of whether the lungs have matured enough to make delivery safe.

Your radiologist will use the ultrasound images to make informed guesses about how far along your fetus's development has come, and how much he or she weighs. These determinations are very important when a decision has to be made about whether or not to deliver the baby.

"It's hard to be completely accurate about the baby's weight," says Dr. Blatman. "It's like trying to guess how much someone weighs just by looking at a picture. But it's the best information we can get."

Another possible complication is known as "failing labor." This means that somewhere along the line, labor stops before the baby comes out.

"There are several ways that this can happen," Dr. Blatman explains. "You may have a situation where cervical dilatation just stops. You may have someone who never gets out of the labor phase. You can fail labor at just about any point along the way. We try to keep a very close watch on our mothers with diabetes so that if any of these complications crop up, we can get on top of it right away and make a decision to do a cesarean, or take whatever action we have to." For a mother with diabetes, it can be extremely comforting to have an experienced high-risk obstetrician there, just in case any complications occur.

If you've followed good medical advice throughout your pregnancy and kept your blood glucose in the prescribed range, chances are very good that after about thirty-eight weeks of pregnancy, you will be thinking about having your baby very soon. The last few weeks may seem like an eternity. Although more and more pregnant women with diabetes are having vaginal deliveries, the rate of cesarean section remains higher than in the nondiabetic population. Although you may have read that too many cesarean deliveries are performed in the U.S., in the setting of diabetic pregnancies they are usually done for very good reasons.

You can expect much more intensive monitoring, including glucose monitoring during labor and delivery. Interestingly, after the progressive increase in your body's insulin requirements during the third trimester, those requirements fall to near zero during active labor. They'll remain low for the first few days after delivery and eventually return to pre-pregnancy levels.

After Delivery

Your new family member will receive extra attention after delivery. Some babies born to mothers with diabetes are somewhat sluggish the first few minutes after delivery. As a consequence, they may score low on the APGAR scale, a measure of fetal activity that is made at the moment of delivery, and then again ten minutes later. The APGAR takes into account the baby's strength, activity, alertness, and appearance. It's not unusual for the baby of a diabetic mother to score a little low on the initial APGAR, but it usually bounces right back by the second one. The initial lower score may not indicate any problem, but rather reflects the baby's size and the stress of labor.

Some mothers with diabetes are surprised when, a few minutes after delivery, their babies are taken to the NICU for observation. Many mothers are understandably distressed, especially because they've taken such pains to have a healthy baby. The close monitoring has a very good medical explanation. If your baby's lungs are still immature at the time of delivery, he or she may need supplemental oxygen, lung treatment, and close observation.

In addition, while your baby was growing inside you, it lived in a relatively nutrient-rich environment. Although your diabetes may have been in very good control, your blood sugar was probably at least intermittently higher than that of a mother without diabetes. Consequently, the baby's pancreas had to produce greater-than-usual amounts of insulin to keep the baby's own blood sugar under control. Your baby comes out of this sugar-rich environment with a pancreas that has an abundance of insulin-producing beta cells. Because the pancreas may leak a little of this insulin after delivery, when the baby may not yet be nursing, the newborn runs a risk of developing hypoglycemia (low blood sugar). In the NICU, nurses will regularly monitor your baby's blood sugar, while they keep 24-hour watch over his or her blood pressure, heart rate, and respiration.

This can be a traumatic time for many mothers. No one likes to see her child in an intensive care unit, no matter how healthy he or she might be. Many mothers with diabetes resent that their babies are so far from them, while they see other mothers in the maternity ward cuddling their newborns.

"It was very hard for me, especially with my first child," says Joan, who was introduced at the beginning of this chapter. "I had decided to breastfeed my baby, and hours after Hanna was born, my breasts became very engorged with milk. At the same time, they were giving Hanna formula in the NICU to make sure that her sugars didn't get too low. I was so engorged and we were both so inexperienced with breastfeeding that it made it very difficult for her to latch on. It took quite a while for both of us to get on the same page, but somehow we did it."

The issue of breastfeeding is very personal to some mothers. Sometimes there may be misunderstandings around this time that can drive a wedge between doctors and patients, as Carmella Clark told me.

"I had Jessie at a hospital near my home in Long Island," she recalls. "She was born hypoglycemic, and she went directly into intensive care. I wanted to breastfeed her, and I could see the nurses bringing babies to all the other mothers on the floor who were breastfeeding. I told my doctor that I had decided to breastfeed Jessie, and he told me that I couldn't because they wanted an accurate measurement of how much she was eating. I was very upset. I had to fight with them to breastfeed, and I couldn't wait to go home."

Your experience need not be like this. During your pregnancy, make it a point to talk with your diabetologist and pediatrician about breastfeeding, and make sure that you come to an understanding with them about what their recommendations will be and what *your* desires are.

As has been said so often, pregnancy is not a disease, and while diabetes may make pregnancy and delivery less carefree than usual, it need not be a painful experience. To make your pregnancy and delivery as joyful and rewarding a time as possible, make sure that you communicate honestly with all the members of your treatment team, and that all your questions about pregnancy and infancy are answered.

Now that your baby has been born, you may wonder what his or her chances are of developing diabetes like you. Diabetes is, to some extent, inherited. Keep in mind that IDDM is relatively rare, affecting only 4 of 1,000 individuals over a lifetime. The risk of your child developing IDDM is increased if you, your husband, or your other children have it. If you have IDDM, the risk increases approximately fivefold, to 2 in 100 (2 percent). If the baby's father also has IDDM, the risk increases even more, about ten- to twentyfold, to 4 to 12 in 100 (4 to 12 percent). The average risk for the child or sibling of a person with

IDDM is probably 5 percent. So even though diabetes is inherited, the chance that your child will have IDDM is relatively small. When parents who are planning a family ask me for my advice regarding their children's chances, I tell them that the *relative* risk is greater than for children of nondiabetic parents, but the *absolute* risk remains low.

Gestational Diabetes Mellitus

As I mentioned earlier, approximately 3 to 5 percent of women who did not have diabetes before they became pregnant develop gestational diabetes mellitus (GDM) during the latter stages of pregnancy. Although GDM is seldom a life-threatening condition and is not associated with an increased risk for birth defects, it is nonetheless serious and demands attention and hard work from the mother to make sure that it does not cause any harm to the baby.

GDM occurs for several reasons. During the last trimester of pregnancy, whether you are diabetic or not, your need for insulin increases. This is partially a result of your increased body mass. In addition, the placenta, an organ that develops during pregnancy to nourish the fetus, releases substances that blunt the effects of insulin. When you're pregnant, your pancreas has to produce more insulin to compensate for these anti-insulin effects. If your pancreas cannot keep up with the demand for extra insulin, which increases as your pregnancy progresses, then you may develop GDM.

Although overweight women over the age of twenty-five or those who have a family history of NIDDM are more likely to develop GDM, there is really no way of predicting exactly who will be affected. However, women who have had an episode of GDM during a previous pregnancy are at increased risk of developing GDM in subsequent pregnancies.

All women should have a screening for GDM during the 24th to the 28th week of pregnancy, unless some reason to suspect GDM arises earlier than that—for example, if you have had GDM during previous pregnancies your physician will want to test you earlier in your pregnancy. The screening procedure—called a *glucose tolerance test*—is quite simple. You'll be given 50 grams of pure glucose, usually in liquid form. If blood glucose monitoring one hour later reveals a blood sugar level of 140 mg/dl or higher, another, more definitive test, using a higher dose (100 grams) of glucose and two blood sugar measurements, will be administered to confirm the diagnosis of GDM. The majority of women who have positive screening tests will prove *not* to have GDM on the more definitive test. You shouldn't be overly concerned if your doctor calls you to come in for the second test, but you shouldn't miss it, either.

If GDM is diagnosed, it's important to address it immediately, because it can lead to some of the same complications with delivery that I outlined earlier in this chapter. First of all, there's a chance that your child will have an abnormally high birth weight, which can present problems during delivery and may require a cesarean section. Also, the baby's lungs may be slower to mature, raising the risk of respiratory distress. There's also the risk of hypoglycemia in your baby right after delivery, which may require a short stay in the NICU.

There are usually no risks for the mother during pregnancy. If you are diagnosed with GDM, you will find that your treatment may require only a change in diet, although you may also need exercise and insulin. The blood sugar goals are the same as those for other diabetic women during pregnancy. Some women with GDM may need insulin from the time of diagnosis, whereas others may need insulin added to their diet and an exercise regimen as they near the end of pregnancy. If you do need insulin, you will probably take it once or twice a day. You'll need to monitor your glucose. Oral agents, such as sulfonylureas and metformin, are generally not an option for women with GDM.

As I mentioned, GDM almost always resolves after delivery, except for the few women who develop IDDM coincidentally during their pregnancy.

In a sense, pregnancy represents a stress test for the insulin-producing beta cells of your pancreas. Women whose insulin-secreting capacity can't keep up with the increased requirements during pregnancy develop GDM. It should come as no surprise that if you have GDM, you are at higher risk for developing NIDDM later in life. Approximately 35 to 50 percent of patients with GDM will develop NIDDM within five to twenty years of their GDM episode. This often happens if their insulin requirements have increased over time from weight gain. Women who have had GDM should pay special attention to their diets and try to avoid excessive weight gain. I recommend that you have annual checkups that include blood tests to make sure that you haven't developed diabetes.

10

Special Considerations for Non-Insulin-Dependent Diabetes Mellitus (NIDDM)

As we discussed in Chapter 1, the differences between insulin-dependent diabetes mellitus (IDDM) and non-insulin-dependent diabetes mellitus (NIDDM), especially with regard to their causes, are so great that they could be regarded as two different diseases. Both diseases cause high blood sugar levels and similar long-term complications. Beyond this point, however, the two conditions diverge in many ways. A major distinction is that NIDDM is almost always associated with obesity: approximately 80 percent of all people with NIDDM are clinically overweight. In addition, people with NIDDM often have high blood pressure and abnormal blood lipid (cholesterol) levels. Another distinguishing feature of NIDDM is something called *insulin resistance*. This means that insulin has less effect in people with NIDDM than in the general population; in other words, a person who is not insulin resistant may need four units of insulin to lower his or her blood sugar by 50 mg/dl, but an insulin-resistant person may need 10 or 20 units to do the same job.

Any one of these conditions—diabetes, insulin resistance, high blood pressure, obesity, or abnormal lipids—increases the risk for heart disease. When they occur together, as is often the case with NIDDM, the risk for heart disease is greatly increased. Since the combination of risk factors above is unusual in people with IDDM, they have a much lower risk for cardiovascular complications, particularly coronary artery disease, than people with NIDDM. A major feature of NIDDM care is to decrease the likelihood for cardiovascular disease by aggressively treating the risk factors.

There are other differences, too. For instance, people with IDDM are at risk of diabetic ketoacidosis (see Chapter 1), whereas people with NIDDM rarely have trouble with this condition. This is because people with NIDDM produce some insulin on their own; in contrast, people with IDDM usually produce no insulin and are totally dependent on the insulin they administer.

The First Line of Treatment: Diet

All these differences between IDDM and NIDDM help explain why treatments for these two diseases also differ considerably. IDDM is basically a *deficiency* of insulin, which is treated by replacing insulin in normal (or *physiologic*) amounts. In IDDM treatment, diet and exercise are regulated and monitored and insulin is adjusted to keep blood sugar levels under control.

NIDDM, on the other hand, is much more closely linked to obesity. When anyone gains weight, they eat more calories in a single day than they can burn up. The extra nourishment is stored as fat, which strains the pancreatic islet, because now they have to produce more insulin to overcome the insulin resistance. Losing weight reverses the insulin resistance. Therefore, in the vast majority of cases, the most important, first order of business in NIDDM treatment is that of diet: *limiting calories to lose weight*. This means eating less of almost everything, particularly sweet and fatty foods that pack a lot of calories.

So your first concern with treating NIDDM if you are overweight is controlling your weight. If I were able to help all my NIDDM patients bring their weight down to an acceptable range, it would erase much of their blood sugar problem. Without their excess weight, many of my patients probably wouldn't need sugar-lowering medications.

Unfortunately, several conditions conspire to make the goal of weight loss difficult to attain. The most obvious problem is cultural. People hesitate to alter their eating habits; in fact, the idea of eating less usually makes people profoundly uncomfortable, simply because eating is often something we do to make ourselves feel secure and happy. Eating is a reward that we all look forward to, no matter who we are or where we live. Deeply ingrained in all cultures is a respect, even a reverence, for food and for eating. It's generally considered a good thing to eat more, not less. (Just take a look at the "buffet night" at your local restaurant, if you doubt how much we emphasize the amounts we eat. Or consider how restaurants advertise their twenty-four- or forty-eight-ounce prime ribs with a guarantee that you can have a free second serving if you finish the first helping without exploding.)

Genetic factors also come into play. Certain people appear to have a genetic predisposition to weight gain. In addition, there are very likely genes that make people vulnerable to NIDDM. Granted, people who have these genes can still lose weight if they work hard at it, but it may be more difficult for them than for other people.

Added to these obstacles to weight loss are many personal, psychological, and other issues that make it difficult for people to lose weight. Many overweight people eat more when they are under stress. In addition, high-fat, high-sugar food is widely available and relatively inexpensive. Despite the introduction of salad bars at the national burger chains, it's the fat-saturated burgers, fries, chicken, and shakes that they advertise and sell the most. Obtaining food is as easy as putting some change into a candy machine or turning off the television, driving to the drive-through window, and ordering. This requires very little effort and little energy is expended. Very few of us work for hours in the fields to harvest the food we eat, or hunt for days to procure meat. Our "hunting" usually involves calling information for the pizza delivery phone number.

Some of the roadblocks to losing weight are put there by our own bodies. Even if you lower your daily calorie intake significantly, another problem occurs, which is related to your metabolism. As was mentioned earlier, your rate of metabolism is the pace at which your body uses energy. If you have a high rate of metabolism, you burn calories faster, and your weight is easier to keep down; if your rate of metabolism is low, it takes you longer to burn up the calories from your food, and they're more likely to be stored as fat.

Whether your natural rate of metabolism is high or low, it is never stable. Changes in your diet and lifestyle can affect your metabolic rate dramatically. Exercise, for instance, speeds metabolism, not just while you're exercising, but the whole day long, so you're always burning more calories than you would be if you didn't exercise. Your age is another factor. As you grow older, you burn fewer calories.

Another thing that affects rate of metabolism is calorie intake and weight. As you eat less food and begin to lose weight, your metabolism slows down to "defend" your weight. It's a normal reaction from the body that, in days long ago when the food supply was inconsistent, probably helped us to avoid starvation during lean times. When you're trying to lose weight by dieting, however, it becomes a problem when your metabolic rate slows each time you make significant reductions in your calorie intake. What this may mean is that you have to increase your metabolic rate deliberately to overwhelm your body's defensive response to your new, lower-calorie diet.

This is exactly what Dan Greenblatt had to do when he was diagnosed with diabetes in his mid-thirties. At age thirty-five, Dan weighed 280 pounds and already had a problem with high blood sugars and insulin resistance. His mother had suffered from complications of diabetes, and Dan decided that, if he wanted to live a long, productive life, he would have to take it upon himself to try to avoid the same thing happening to him. Dan took the challenge seriously, cutting back on sweets and limiting the amount of food he ate at meals. He cut his intake of calories drastically. At one point, he even kept himself to a low-fat and low-calorie macrobiotic diet for almost a year. He also ran two to three miles every day, to increase his metabolic rate. He built up his endurance until, by his fortieth birthday, he was able to run five miles daily.

"I got my blood sugar under such good control that I

got a few of my doctors to join the program, too," he told me.

After many years of dietary treatment, however, Dan found that in order to keep his blood sugar in a healthy range, he needed to start taking insulin. We find that a fairly high proportion of the people we treat for NIDDM need to start taking insulin eventually. This need for insulin is often because people regain the weight they lost or just because they have aged. Both instances increase their insulin resistance. Some NIDDM patients start taking insulin when they're first diagnosed with diabetes, and most adjust to it relatively quickly and easily. However, there is one difficulty that occurs when people begin controlling their blood sugar with insulin or sulfonylureas (pills that lower blood sugar levels by stimulating insulin secretion): they *gain* weight.

It sounds paradoxical at first, but it makes sense. When the amount of insulin you have on board is inadequate, sugar stays in the bloodstream rather than being absorbed into fat and skeletal tissues. (These high blood sugars, if left uncorrected, will later cause complications.) Some of the sugar is lost in your urine. As a result, you lose weight, or gain it more slowly than you would otherwise. (Some people are diagnosed with NIDDM when they begin to lose weight for no apparent reason.)

When you start taking insulin, you remove that excess sugar from your circulation, protecting your eyes, kidneys, nerves, and other tissues from the damage that high blood sugar levels can cause. The amount of sugar in your urine decreases. Instead of "spilling" sugar and calories into the toilet, you now absorb those calories. The sugar is absorbed by fat and skeletal cells and you begin to gain or at least maintain weight.

Whether you have diabetes or not, losing weight—or changing your diet in any way—is no easy task. No physician, dietitian, or diet guru can order you up a foolproof weight-loss program. There are always challenges, snags, breakdowns, losses of will, increases in appetite. A myriad of things can and will go wrong, despite your best efforts to lose weight.

The first step in approaching a healthy diet is to determine your usual eating habits. I encourage my patients to talk frankly and openly with their treatment team here at Mass General and with family members about their eating habits. All of us have the same goal: to encourage the person with diabetes to continue living a productive, healthy, and satisfying life. Eating is part of everyday life, and it should be a centerpiece of healthy living. No one can hide what they eat and enjoy life at the same time. Acceptance of your diet is an important part of accepting yourself as a person.

A dietitian can be particularly helpful in helping you understand your eating habits and making them more manageable for you. Many overweight people have problems with snacking, binge eating, and eating certain foods that make blood sugar go higher. A dietitian can help you spot these problem-eating behaviors and suggest solutions.

Mass General dietitian Linda Delahanty and I often talk about how we can best work with patients to help them control their weight and their eating habits. We both know that it isn't necessary that patients lose a lot of weight to get their blood sugar under control. In some people with NIDDM, blood sugar normalizes after they lose only two or three pounds.

That's right; sometimes as little as two or three pounds can make the difference between your pancreas providing adequate insulin or your blood sugar running out of control. Sometimes it's more. When I begin talking with patients about weight control, they often anticipate that I'll ask them to go on a starvation diet, and that they'll have to give up all their favorite foods. They soon relax when they see the actual objectives.

When I refer a patient to Linda, the first thing she does is find out what he or she is eating and when. Initially, each patient must give Linda a very quick "food diary," a description of a typical day of eating, usually from their recall of the previous day's menu. Linda uses this information to determine how many calories the patient is eating, how much in grams of fat, how much in carbohydrates, in protein, and in fiber.

Linda also takes a close look at what time of day patients get their calories. For instance, we have had several patients come through our clinic with NIDDM who were not severely overweight, but nonetheless they had high blood sugars at certain times of day. Upon taking a diet history, Linda found that these people normally skipped breakfast and lunch. They were very busy at their offices during the day, and preferred to eat a big dinner and then snack liberally before going to bed. In these cases, the high load of nutrients converted to blood sugar at one time of the day had overmatched the pancreas's ability to crank out insulin. In addition, eating all of your calories at one meal tends to lower your metabolic rate (the rate at which you burn off calories) and will predispose you to gain more weight, compared to spreading your calories throughout the day. Linda's solution was to instruct these patients to begin eating some breakfast and lunch, to go a little bit easier at dinner, and to reduce the snacking after dinner. Relieving the high load of carbohydrate at dinner and before bedtime spread out their blood sugar load, and the pancreas was able to keep up.

After taking the diet history, Linda takes the number of calories and compares that to an estimate of the number of calories the patient would need to maintain his or her current weight. For instance, with my current height, weight, sex, age, and activity level, I need about 2,500 calories per day to maintain my weight. If I eat substantially more than that over a long period of time, I'll start to gain pounds; if I eat less, I'll shed them.

Once she has an idea of what the patient is taking in, Linda can begin looking for ways to create constructive, lasting changes in the diet. She makes a point of targeting what she calls "liquid carbohydrates," such as fruit juice and regular sodas. A regular twelve-ounce cola packs about 160 calories. That's a lot, considering you can get almost the same taste from a diet cola, while consuming only one calorie. High-sugar foods like this can have a tremendous impact on blood sugar over the course of a day, so naturally Linda tries to make sure that all our patients drink only diet soft drinks, and that they drink fruit juices in limited quantities to counteract hypoglycemia (see Chapter 7).

Taking the diet history is an ongoing process. A dietitian can't find out everything about your diet in just one visit. People have favorite tastes that they infrequently indulge, they may have eating habits that they keep secret from other people, and they themselves may not be aware of how much they are snacking during a typical day. It takes time for a dietitian to find out as much as he or she can about what, how, and when you eat, and to help you understand the effect that your eating pattern has on your weight and blood sugar levels. I asked Linda to describe how she would approach treating me if I were eating substantially more than what I needed to maintain my desired weight.

"A lot depends on what kind of person you are," she replied. "Because you're a 'numbers' person—someone who likes to think in terms of facts and figures, so to speak—I would probably try to get you to count your calories. We would spend a little time with a chart that shows how many calories are found in different foods, like milk, bread, eggs, fruit. You would take the chart home and start using it to add up your calorie intake for each day of the week. Your weekend intake might be completely different from days that you're at work.

"This would help educate you about how the food you eat affects your blood sugar levels. If you were treated with insulin, for example, and were keeping track of your blood sugar levels, I'd be able to show you how the food you eat raises and lowers your blood sugars from hour to hour, and day to day.

"For instance, we could start talking about how foods in different forms affect your blood sugars. We know that fruit is a very good food choice for people with diabetes, because in addition to its good flavor, it's relatively low in sugar, high in fiber, and totally fat free. But there's a huge difference between eating fruit and drinking fruit juice, which is full of concentrated sugar that is absorbed quickly from your intestine and can quickly cause your blood sugar to spike. Canned fruit is also much more sugary than raw fruit. For instance, a pear has about 100 calories in it, but one cup of canned pears in syrup has 195 calories. These distinctions are very important when it comes to controlling your weight and your blood sugar.

"After we've made some progress there, we can start paying attention to how many calories you consume in the form of carbohydrate, fat, and protein. (For an explanation of how to read food labels, see Chapter 4.) This is important because these three forms of food contribute to weight in very different ways. As you know, fatty foods are very concentrated in calories and raise lipid levels, which in turn leads to heart disease. So naturally we would try to find some ways to reduce the fat in your diet. For instance, if you eat toast with butter every day, I might try to get you to eat an all-fruit, naturally sweetened jam instead of butter on your bread because it's lower in both fat *and* calories. So if you start making that substitution in a routine manner, it can make a real difference in your diet, in your weight, and in your blood sugar numbers."

Linda's hardest and most important job is getting people to stick—*really* stick—with the dietary changes she asks them to make. For this reason, she tries never to ask too much of a person at any one time. To her, it's more important that her patients understand why they're making certain changes, recognize the consequences of failing to make them, and see the good results of maintaining the dietary alterations that she and the patient have decided on.

"Change often comes slowly," she says, "but that's the nature of lasting change. One of my patients came in last week and said she was disappointed in herself because she'd lost "only" one pound in two weeks. 'I could have lost more,' she said. In this country, we all want to do everything right away, it seems. Anyway, I agreed with her that one pound didn't look like very much at the time, but that if she was able to keep up that pace, she would have lost twenty-six pounds over the year. And we both agreed that that would be terrific.

"Another patient of mine came in gaining weight at a terrific rate after he stopped smoking. When we began working together, he became disappointed because he wasn't losing weight right away. I pointed out to him that his blood sugars had normalized, and he had stopped gaining weight. Those were both very important things to do, and they took a lot of work, and I tried to let him know that I was very pleased with his progress. He had stopped smoking, a very important step. Each week, we work on doing *something* to reduce the fat and overall calories in his diet, and each change we've made so far has been permanent. And that's extremely important when you're dealing with diet, because old dietary habits are the hardest things to break."

Some of Linda's patients find it hard to be precise about numbers, and they have a hard time counting calories. So for them, Linda is more likely to start giving them printed diets that they can follow from day to day. Other good sources of dietary information are the American Diabetes Association's publication *Diabetes Forecast* and the magazine *Diabetes Self-Management,* both of which regularly publish recipes and diets for people with IDDM and NIDDM. For instance, here's a 1,500-calorie meal plan from the American Dietetic Association's *Meal-Planning Approaches for Diabetes Management.*

BREAKFAST:
1 cup skim milk or 1 cup sugar-free non-fat yogurt
½ banana or ½ grapefruit or 2 tablespoons of raisins
2 slices of toast or 1 bagel or 1 cup hot cereal
1 egg or 1 oz. of low-fat cheese
1 teaspoon of margarine or 2 tablespoons of cream
  cheese

LUNCH:
Green salad with fat-free dressing or 4 oz. low-sodium
   vegetable juice
1 pear or 1 orange or 1 apple
2 slices of bread or 1 roll or 10 melba toast triangles
2 oz. of lean beef, poultry, or fish, or ½ cup tuna or
   ½ cup cottage cheese
1 teaspoon mayonnaise or 1 tablespoon salad dressing

DINNER:
Green salad with fat-free dressing
1 cup green vegetables
½ cup applesauce or 1 cup cubed melon
1 large potato or ½ cup corn or 1½ cup pasta or 1 cup
   rice
2 oz. lean meat, poultry, or fish, or 4 oz. shellfish
2 teaspoons oil or margarine

BEDTIME SNACK:
¾ cup cereal or 1 Dutch pretzel or 3 graham crackers
4 oz. skim milk

This particular menu offers about 1,500 calories, yet a little less than a third of them come from fat. As we mentioned
before, keeping fat to a minimum is of great importance for
people with NIDDM. People who like menus like this appreciate simplicity. It doesn't require too much thought to
choose between applesauce and melon or between poultry
and fish. This is just the "skeleton" of a diet (no, it won't
turn you into a skeleton) that provides basic nutrition. In
consultation with a dietitian, you can easily work in snacks
and other supplemental foods that will take care of your
specific nutritional (and emotional) needs.

On the other hand, it may be difficult to follow a menu like this if you have an erratic daily schedule that prevents you from eating three meals a day. Lots of people find themselves in meetings at times of day when their dietitians think they ought to be eating or snacking. If you have an erratic eating schedule, but could accommodate more order in your life, then menu planning might be just what you need to get your eating habits under control. Consultation with your dietitian will help you decide whether this approach is right for you.

Some people find they have more success with a menu-planning approach when they use a planning tool called "Month of Meals." Each of the four books in the "Month of Meals" series contains twenty-eight full-day 1500-calorie menus. The menus can be adjusted to provide slightly more or fewer calories, depending on the need of the individual. Snack menus are included.

Linda and I talked about what happens when patients break their diets, either by consuming more calories than they're supposed to, or by reverting to high-fat foods. First of all, Linda pointed out, she can almost always find a difference in blood sugar readings, if the patient has been monitoring regularly, depending on food intake. Pointing out those differences helps motivate patients to eat fewer sweets and avoid fat in their diets.

Because it occurs so often in older people, NIDDM is frequently complicated by other conditions, particularly heart disease. The first thing cardiologists often discuss with their patients with heart disease is the necessity of changing their diets in order to lose weight and minimize fat and cholesterol. If you have diabetes and heart disease, you may well have to listen to two doctors giving separate instructions about how to deal with your diet. A diet high in fat, especially saturated fat, can create high levels of cholesterol in the bloodstream, which predisposes people to heart disease. So, just like your diabetes diet, your healthy-heart diet is likely to require that you cut lots of fat out of your meals and snacks.

Although a healthy-heart diet and a diabetes diet have much in common, the pressure of having to conform to a very strict diet may create problems for you. You might feel trapped, as though there's nothing you can eat, that you're deprived of an important part of your life, one that you enjoy. "I don't have any choice," some patients tell me. "I have to eat *something*." A feeling of futility often leads people to think that they can't avoid going back to their accustomed diet. I talked with Martin Cohen, a patient with both diabetes and heart disease, about this problem, and he expressed some very familiar concerns.

"For my heart there is food I cannot eat, and for my diabetes there is food I cannot eat," he says. "Consequently there is very little that I *can* eat."

I asked Martin how he copes with this feeling that there's nothing for him to eat that's within his diet.

"What do you do? You cheat. Will I eat a scoop of ice cream? Yes. Will I eat a candy bar or two or three if I feel a low coming on? Yes."

Needless to say, I sympathize with everyone who feels that they are trapped by their diet regimen and recognize that almost everyone "cheats." The challenge for Martin and others is to make digressions from your diet plan the exception and not the rule. Try to stick to your plan *most* of the time and if you find yourself less than perfect on occasion, or even on many occasions, don't get frustrated and give up. Do the best you can. If you take insulin and are experienced enough, you can usually compensate for the effect that dietary "adventures" will have on your blood sugar by changing your insulin dose. You may even be able to counteract some dietary transgressions with exercise.

However, you can't start making positive changes with your diet until you start to understand that there are important reasons for changing your diet, and that failure to make those changes will likely lead to further health problems for you. A good relationship with a dietitian will help you understand the issues and deal with them through knowledge, rather than ignorance. Let's talk more about another very important dimension of dealing with NIDDM: exercise.

Exercise

How would you prefer to care for you diabetes? Would you rather take medications? Or would you rather think of diabetes as a powerful motivator to keep you exercising and eating right?

Lots of people think of diabetes as a curse; you can also think of it as a *coach,* one who requires you to maintain healthy eating habits and a moderate regimen of exercise. The majority of people with NIDDM—as many as 60 to 80 percent—can potentially control their diabetes with diet and/or exercise and never have to use medications. If you would like to be one of those people, read on.

Exercise has always been considered part of diabetes therapy, because it does all kinds of terrific things for you. Let's quickly go down a short list of exercise bonuses:

• Although it hasn't been shown that exercise actually *prevents* NIDDM, many studies indicate that physical activity is associated with an overall *protective effect.* In other words, people who exercise appear less likely to develop NIDDM in the first place.

- Exercise can help you lose weight by raising your metabolic rate. This is a plus for many people who don't have diabetes. But if you have NIDDM, it can have even greater benefits. Many people with NIDDM could reduce or eliminate their dependence on diabetic medications by losing weight. Wouldn't it make your life easier if you could do that?

- Regular exercise can lower your blood pressure and your percentage of body fat, as well as your cholesterol. Decreasing these factors lowers your risk for heart disease, to which people with diabetes are already highly vulnerable. Even light exercise performed regularly will help you avoid this important complication of diabetes.

- Exercise improves cardiovascular "conditioning." Your heart, when conditioned with regular exercise, needs to work less for a given amount of activity. This relieves stress on the heart muscle and improves the circulation.

- Exercise increases your insulin sensitivity. Whether you have IDDM or NIDDM, exercise will reduce your insulin requirements.

- Exercise can be a great way to meet other people.

- Exercise helps relieve stress, which is another risk factor for heart disease. Regular exercise also discourages people from smoking, and quitting smoking gives even more protection from heart disease.

- Some people claim that exercise dulls the appetite for random snacking (it's hard to eat *while* you're jogging or swimming). Many people also find that exercise helps clear their heads, and it puts them in a better frame of mind. It can give you motivation to take care of other tasks, such as managing your diabetes.

- Exercise is another way to reassert control over your life.

And that's just a short list. If you heard of a pill that would do all these things for you, you would comb the shelves of your drugstore to find it. Exercise can do all this, and it's virtually FREE! The biggest investment you make is time.

Of course, NIDDM tends to occur in older people, and many people with NIDDM suffer from complicating conditions. People with NIDDM often have to be conscientious about caring for themselves because of the major complications of diabetes—eye disease, kidney disease, heart disease, neuropathy, and foot problems. At the same time, they may be suffering from other, related problems, such as high blood pressure and obesity, and unrelated problems like osteoporosis, cancer, or respiratory disease. Consequently, for many people with NIDDM, exercise looks like a very risky proposition. It's very important to have the attention and approval of your doctor before embarking on any kind of an exercise program. You may find that your doctor can point you toward a facility where the exercise specialists on the staff know all about diabetes and how to prevent and treat low blood sugars. It's much safer and easier to exercise if you're working with someone who understands that you're not trying to fit into a bathing suit: you're just trying to fit your blood sugar into a healthy range!

Doctors and exercise specialists recommend exercise for their patients for a number of important reasons: its positive effect on weight, the benefits it provides for heart health, the prevention of complications and other diseases, not to mention the fact that exercise often makes people feel better and happier. But the most important reason is that, in people whose blood glucose elevation is mild or moderate, exercise can keep blood sugar in or close to a healthy range.

What's more, the effects of exercise stay with you. Even after you've finished working out, exercise continues to act somewhat like insulin, reducing your blood sugar for at least a few hours afterwards, and sometimes longer. Exercise also reduces your resistance to insulin; as we discussed in Chapter 1, one of the causes behind NIDDM is that your cells have become less responsive to insulin. Exercise appears to restore some of that sensitivity, thereby reducing your need for medications.

So exercise is a priority for treating NIDDM. First of all, though, you and your treatment team have to evaluate your potential to exercise safely. Exercise is like a drug in that it has certain potential side effects, but they can be foreseen and controlled. Vigorous exercise may cause irregular heartbeat and some increases in blood pressure. If you take insulin or sulfonylureas and your blood sugar is low before exercising, you could suffer hypoglycemia while exercising; paradoxically, sometimes exercise may *raise* blood sugar and even lead to a life-threatening condition called diabetic ketoacidosis (see Chapter 1). However, if you have NIDDM, this is much less a risk for you than it would be for someone with IDDM. Remember, if you take insulin check your blood sugar before you exercise, and definitely after you've finished working out. If your blood sugar is low before you start, you may need a snack to prevent it from falling more. You may also want to monitor your blood sugar a couple of hours after you've finished exercising, to avoid lingering lows.

Exercise has other dangers that affect people with diabetes, as well as those without the disease. The pounding of aerobic exercise sometimes aggravates existing injuries. If you have NIDDM, you should be checked for neuropathy before beginning a new exercise regimen, and seek your doctor's advice about how to avoid inflicting damage to your feet. There's also the risk of eye damage to be considered, and of course people with diabetes have to guard their eyes very carefully (see Chapter 6). Even an easy round of calisthenics can place unforeseen stress on different parts of the body. Exertion dilates blood vessels, quick movements load extra weight onto joints, bones, and tendons, and pulling and pushing fatigues muscles.

Consequently, it's important to get a thorough physical before starting an exercise program. Your doctor should check you for heart disease and neurological complications, diabetic eye disease, kidney disease, and foot ulcers. You should also speak openly with your doctor or diabetes educator about your plans and goals for exercise. Let him or her know how much exercise and the type of exercise you would like to do, and how much weight you expect to lose as a result.

Unfortunately, many people feel daunted by exercise, unsure that they want to go to the trouble of learning how to master it. At Mass General we try to provide motivation for people by showing them how far their blood sugar levels drop after just a few minutes of moderate exercise. I watched Meryl Cohen as she had some of her "students" test their blood sugar just before and then again just after exercising. Some were amazed at the reductions they could achieve in only fifteen minutes of walking on a treadmill or riding on a stationary bike.

"People are always surprised at how they can lower their blood sugars with exercising," Meryl said when we sat down to talk for a few minutes. "Most of them are very impressed and satisfied with the results, and they're glad that they tried it. The main problem that we have is getting people to stick with the program. It can be extremely difficult to motivate some patients to keep up an exercise program."

Some patients don't realize all the exercise options that are open to them. For instance, some of my patients who are worried about the impact and exertion of running or walking have tried relatively low-impact exercise, like yoga. One patient has been able to halve her daily sulfonylurea dose with a six-days-a-week yoga program. The yoga classes are ninety minutes long, but she's very happy with the results and with the fact that she's avoided going onto an insulin regimen. "You can't imagine how I feel when I walk out of class," she says. "I feel like a million dollars, tax free." Other forms of low-impact exercise include swimming, biking, and walking. I particularly encourage walking because almost anyone can do it, anytime, anywhere. There's nothing competitive about it, and no technique is involved. If you have difficulty walking and are looking for other ways of getting some exercise, consult an exercise therapist and see what suggestions he or she has for your particular case.

Medications

If you have NIDDM, that means you're not dependent on insulin. Of course, *dependent* is a relative term (my children prove that to me every day). If you have NIDDM and use insulin every day, you might think to yourself, "Well, I *depend* on insulin; I use it every day!" But with NIDDM, you have other treatment and medication options for keeping your blood sugar under control, options that people with IDDM don't have. Moreover, if you stop your insulin you won't die, which is likely to happen if an IDDM patient stops.

We've already talked about two important options: diet and exercise. These will continue to be the "front line" of your battle with NIDDM. If you don't control your diet and don't make use of whatever ability you may have to perform some kind of exercise, your diabetes will be that much harder to control. Even if you do begin taking blood-sugar-lowering medications, you'll still need to continue your regimen of reduced-calorie and low-fat meals. If you have NIDDM, you will probably need to regulate your dietary habits in this way for the rest of your life, making sure to eat balanced meals at more or less regular times. This will go a long way toward making your blood sugar control easier.

If and when you do start taking medications—sometimes called *hypoglycemics* because they keep blood sugar down—it will probably come about only after you and your doctor have made an attempt to control your blood sugar with diet and/or exercise. Medications can help control your blood sugar, but they can't do the whole job. The farther you get from your exercise and diet objectives, the more hypoglycemic medication you'll have to take. And the more medication you take, the more likely it is that you'll have to begin taking insulin at some point.

Why is this? A look at the different hypoglycemic medications and what they do will help explain why you need to keep your weight and diet under control, even if you use medications to help control your blood sugar. If you have tried unsuccessfully to manage your diabetes with diet and exercise, your doctor will probably suggest that you begin taking one of several types of medications: a sulfonylurea, metformin, acarbose, insulin, or even a combination of them.

Sulfonylureas

Sulfonylureas, such as glipizide (Glucotrol) and glyburide (Micronase and Diabeta), are among the most commonly prescribed oral medications used to treat diabetes. Most patients with NIDDM who "fail" dietary therapy—meaning that their blood sugar control is not acceptable—and who need a medication would prefer to take a pill rather than an insulin injection. However, there are limitations to these drugs. Sulfonylureas are a group of drugs that were discovered accidently during the development of the sulfa antibiotics more than fifty years ago. They lower blood sugar by stimulating your pancreas to make more insulin. Since people with IDDM are incapable of making their own insulin, and some patients with NIDDM, especially the thin ones, make very little insulin, the sulfonylureas don't work in those patients. They do lower blood sugar levels moderately in the majority of overweight persons with NIDDM. By moderately, I mean that if you continue your dietary efforts and take sulfonylureas, they will probably lower your sugar levels to an acceptable range, although they are unlikely to stabilize them for a sustained amount of time.

Unfortunately, for reasons that are not well understood, sulfonylureas don't work in about 10 to 20 percent of NIDDM patients who try them. In addition, they stop being effective in about 10 percent of NIDDM patients per year. Therefore, by the end of five years, the majority of NIDDM patients who have been using sulfonylureas are no longer receiving an acceptable benefit from them, and usually need to be changed to insulin.

In addition to the limitations above, sulfonylureas can cause a variety of side effects, including hypoglycemia, and relatively rare allergic reactions. (If you are allergic to sulfa antibiotics, you shouldn't take this type of hypoglycemic agent.) In the 1960s, a large study called the University Group Diabetes Program (UGDP), suggested a link between the use of sulfonylureas and heart disease. Although this study has never been refuted, sulfonylureas continue to be widely used in the treatment of NIDDM.

Although we at Mass General do prescribe sulfonylureas to selected patients with NIDDM, we do so cautiously, advising the patients that the effectiveness of these drugs is short-lived and that they may require treatment with insulin within the next five to ten years. Most of the sulfonylureas can be given once or twice per day. They are usually started at a low dose and increased based on your response to them. Self-glucose monitoring may be helpful in determining their effectiveness and the need to adjust your dose. Some doctors will combine them with metformin (see below) or insulin therapy, giving an intermediate-acting insulin at bedtime and sulfonylurea in the morning.

Metformin

An existing drug for treatment of NIDDM was recently introduced to the United States when the U.S. Food and Drug Administration approved *metformin,* currently sold under the brand name Glucophage. Metformin, first developed in the 1950s, is one of the most widely used drugs prescribed for NIDDM. Because of its relative safety and effectiveness, this drug promises to be used even more frequently for NIDDM treatment in the years to come. It has several advantages over sulfonylureas that could prove to be very helpful in certain people with NIDDM.

Metformin lowers your blood sugar levels independent of insulin levels. The drug interferes with the release of glucose from your liver. Your liver normally synthesizes and releases sugar into the bloodstream. Metformin gets in the way of this process and lowers blood sugar levels.

Unlike sulfonylureas, metformin is effective in thin and overweight persons with NIDDM. Metformin is about as powerful as sulfonylureas, but also becomes less effective over time. Because metformin and sulfonylureas work in such different ways, they can be combined when treatment with either one fails, with very good results in lowering blood sugar.

Metformin has several other benefits. It does not increase weight the way sulfonylureas and insulin do when they lower blood sugar levels. And a final, very important selling point for metformin is that, unlike sulfonylureas, it does *not* cause hypoglycemia. However, if you're taking sulfonylureas and metformin at the same time, that risk still does exist.

Metformin's chief side effects are gastrointestinal (flatulence, nausea, and diarrhea). These side effects are rarely severe enough to require discontinuing metformin, but doses may need to be decreased. Metformin also presents a very low risk of *lactic acidosis*. This is a potentially fatal condition in which lactic acid enters your bloodstream quickly, changing your body's acid level. Although this is rarely caused by metformin use, it's quite dangerous when it does occur. Patients with abnormal kidney function, or severe heart failure or circulatory problems should never be treated with metformin, since they are at higher risk for this serious complication.

Your doctor will probably prescribe two or three doses of metformin each day. Pills come in 500- and 850-mg sizes. Slowly increasing the dose will decrease the development of gastrointestinal side effects.

Acarbose

A relatively new oral drug with an entirely different mechanism of action from sulfonylureas or metformin has been recently approved for use in the treatment of NIDDM. Acarbose (Precose) is a drug that blocks the absorption of carbohydrate from the intestine by inhibiting the enzyme in the intestine that breaks down dietary carbohydrate. The digestion of dietary carbohydrate is delayed until it travels farther "downstream" in the intestine. As a result, the rise in blood sugar after a meal is blunted, allowing the available insulin to do its job more effectively.

Acarbose is the weakest of the hypoglycemic drugs and may be best suited as a single drug therapy for patients with relatively mild NIDDM. However, because it acts in a unique manner, it can be combined with any of the other agents, lowering sugar levels further. (It may also be effective in lowering blood sugar levels after meals in IDDM.) Acarbose has several appealing features and one unappealing side effect. It is not absorbed from the intestine, and therefore has little in the way of systemic side effects or allergies. However, by delaying the digestion of carbohydrate until it reaches the large intestine, acarbose allows the bacteria in the large intestine to ferment the nutrients, producing intestinal gas with predictable symptoms. This gaseous side effect may prevent as many as 20 to 30 percent of NIDDM patients from continuing to use acarbose. However, for those patients who can continue to take acarbose, it is a safe and effective hypoglycemic medication. Acarbose is given as you start eating each meal.

Doses of either 50 or 100 mg can be used and need to be adjusted based on the results, and side effects, that occur.

Insulin

Many people with diabetes want to wait as long as possible before going on insulin. They associate insulin with unpleasant things, namely needles. The idea of starting each and every day with a shot of insulin often makes people cringe, and they'll do anything they can to avoid it.

At Mass General, we don't think it's such a bad thing for NIDDM patients to take insulin; in fact, we encourage it in many cases. Most people get comfortable with the injections pretty quickly, although there are some who have difficulty with the concept for quite some time. Not surprisingly, many people associate needles with pain and severe illness. They may also be confused by the process of matching their insulin dose to diet and activity (see Chapter 5).

But, as a medication, insulin has many great qualities. It is relatively inexpensive, it lowers blood sugar in a reliable, consistent manner, and if used in sufficiently large doses always lowers blood sugars. There are several different kinds of insulin you can take for different situations, and best of all, in NIDDM it's extremely safe, with rare episodes of severe hypoglycemia.

If you're newly diagnosed with diabetes and have relatively mild blood sugar elevation, your doctor may nonetheless prescribe insulin for you, particularly if you have concurrent health problems that prevent your use of the oral drugs. We often start new NIDDM patients with insulin treatment right from the time they're diagnosed, if we feel that they may not fare well with oral drug treatment for very long. If you are going to have to begin taking insulin within a matter of weeks or months anyway, there's no reason to "protect" you from learning about it. Proper utilization of insulin is a skill, and the sooner you understand how to implement it, the better off you'll be in the long run.

If your doctor prescribes insulin for you, it's not a sign that you are "sicker" than other people with NIDDM. Keep in mind that the most severe health threats of diabetes come in the form of complications, especially heart disease, eye disease, kidney disease, and neuropathy. If your doctor does prescribe insulin, he or she is probably hoping to help you get your blood sugar under control so that you can successfully avoid these complications, or perhaps halt the further development of complications that have already been detected.

Many people with NIDDM follow an insulin program that is quite simple. There is usually no need for the frequent injections or monitoring that I described for IDDM. In NIDDM, the total dose of insulin is probably more important than the number of injections. It has been common practice for many physicians to prescribe one shot a day of some intermediate- or long-acting insulin—NPH, lente, or ultralente—for the entire day. (To review these types of insulin, see Chapter 5.) This kind of one-shot prescription is designed to reduce chronically high blood sugars throughout the day. NPH, lente, or ultralente, work to lower blood sugar for anywhere from eight to twenty-four hours. In NIDDM, one or two daily injections is usually sufficient to control blood sugars in the near-normal range.

Many of our patients take 70/30 insulin—a preparation that is 70 percent intermediate-acting NPH insulin and 30 percent rapid-acting regular insulin. Taking insulin this way means that you get two peaks of activity from one injection: the regular insulin peaks about two hours after the injection, and the NPH peaks about five or six hours after the injection. If you take the mixed insulin before breakfast and eat your lunch about four hours after breakfast, that one shot of insulin should keep your blood sugar under control for both of those meals.

The advantage of using mixed insulin is that it gives you more insulin coverage from just one shot of insulin. NIDDM can also be treated quite effectively with a bedtime dose of NPH or lente, adjusted to lower the fasting blood sugar to between 80 and 140. Sometimes the evening insulin will be sufficient to lower blood sugar throughout the day. For other patients, a morning dose of NPH or 70/30 insulin will need to be added.

For all of these regimens, it is important to use a large enough dose of insulin. Usually, more than 50 units per day, and often more than 100 units are necessary. As with IDDM, glucose monitoring should be used to help adjust doses. Since blood sugar levels are characteristically more stable and consistent in NIDDM than in IDDM, monitoring can usually be performed once to twice per day while doses are adjusted. As with the other drug therapies for NIDDM, it is critical to continue diet and exercise therapy with insulin therapy.

11

The Diabetes Control and Complications Trial: The New Frontier of Diabetes Care

When was the last time you heard the phrase "Four out of five doctors surveyed recommend . . ." on the TV or radio? It makes it sound as though "a survey of doctors" ought to be sufficient to tell you whether or not something relieves headaches or hemorrhoids, fights colds, or helps you cope with diabetes.

Ideally, that's not how decisions are made in the medical field. At its best, medical care is the product of years' worth of knowledge, experience, and investigation. As I mentioned at the beginning of this book, physicians have been studying diabetes since the dawn of recorded history. Countless treatments, diets, exercise programs, and other interventions have been tried; some have worked, some have not. But none of the time spent in diabetes research—following people with diabetes, working with animals with diabetes, or even looking at beta cells in the test tube—has been wasted. It has helped us accumulate a store of knowledge through systematic observations of normal and abnormal biological processes. After a great deal of knowledge about a medical treatment has been collected, the final step is the controlled clinical trial. These trials are the experiments in which therapies are put to the test in humans. Different therapies are compared with regard to their safety, efficacy, and side effects as part of a carefully controlled study in which the results are collected using standardized methods.

A control, or comparison group, is always included so that we can have a basis for judging the outcome. Generally, the control group is treated with the prevailing or conventional therapy and the experimental group is treated with the new therapy. The results can be viewed as relative to the usual therapy—better, worse, or the same. In order to make the comparisons between the treatments as fair as possible, volunteers for such studies are assigned randomly to the different treatment groups. Neither the scientists conducting the trial nor the participants are allowed to choose who receives which therapy. When possible, the investigators and subjects are prevented from knowing which treatment they are receiving and the results of therapy until the end of the study. This is called a *double-blind trial,* and it helps protect against experimental bias or expectations.

As you can imagine, patients play a major role in this process. They are active partners in these studies, following specific therapies, keeping appointments to have research data collected, and, in general, participating in the experiment. Most important, patients who volunteer for such studies commit themselves to advance our knowledge with the hope of improving the treatment available for themselves and others.

The 1,441 people with IDDM who were enrolled in the Diabetes Control and Complications Trial (DCCT) made an extraordinary ten-year commitment to answer one of the most important questions in medicine: Would therapies designed to control blood sugar in the near-normal range prevent development of, and/or slow the progression of, the devastating long-term complications of diabetes?

In order to answer this question, the volunteers agreed to participate in perhaps the most rigorous, detailed, and demanding clinical trial ever performed. After all, not only did the investigators require one half of the people studied to use new methods of diabetes therapy, which included frequent monitoring and injections and intensive attention to diet, exercise, and lifestyle, but everyone in the study had to have numerous and frequent tests performed to follow the development and course of their eye, kidney, nerve, and heart disease, and to track their quality of life, their psychological status, and dozens of other outcomes.

"The DCCT took me out of my workday, to a certain extent," says Ralph Dineen, who switched to an insulin pump for the study. "But I planned for it, just as I do for all the other commitments that I make, so it did not really affect my work negatively."

Ralph joined the DCCT not long after becoming diabetic. He was very interested in keeping his blood sugar under tight control, but he had had no experience with using the pump. Ralph agreed to join the study without knowing to which group he would be assigned. He was assigned to the intensive therapy group and, not long after beginning with the pump, Ralph noticed that he was getting hypoglycemic at certain times of the day, sometimes in business meetings. This is not surprising; hypoglycemic episodes are more common when people with diabetes start controlling their blood sugar more tightly. Rather than look at it as a dire warning, however, Ralph thought of it as a sign of progress.

"I knew that my blood sugars were getting lower, and it was just a question of dealing with the very low blood sugars before I could really say that I was under very good control."

It was the dedication of volunteers like Ralph that allowed the successful completion of the DCCT. The results of the trial have rewritten the standards of diabetes care, probably for the next twenty years. This could not have been accomplished without the extraordinary level of patient cooperation, which surpassed anything that had ever been seen in shorter, less demanding studies. During the ten-year course of the DCCT, less than 1 percent of the study population dropped out. In addition, the two treatment groups stuck to their assigned therapies with remarkable dedication—they followed their complicated therapies more than 97 percent of the time.

The tenacity and devotion of the participants in the DCCT demonstrate two things: (1) intensive therapy can be done; people with IDDM can keep their blood sugar under tight control, if they learn how to do it and are properly supervised; and (2) the results of the study are highly reliable. We know that the participants in the study were doing what they were asked to do, and we know the ranges of their blood sugar levels. It makes it very difficult for anyone to say that the patients in the intensive therapy group were "just lucky," or that there were other factors at work here. *The remarkable achievements of the patients themselves* were crucial in making sure that the study was unassailable, that it was a reflection of fact and not mere conjecture or opinion. I can't say enough about the courage, tenacity, dedication, and spirit of the DCCT volunteers who made it all possible.

Why the DCCT Was Initiated

Before the discovery of insulin, IDDM was a fatal disease. If you had been diagnosed with diabetes in 1920, you probably wouldn't have lived to see 1922.

Then, insulin treatment came along, and the metabolic disorder of IDDM diabetes was suddenly "cured." Whether or not people could keep their blood sugars in a normal, nondiabetic range didn't seem important at the time. Children and young adults who would previously have been given a death sentence with the diagnosis of diabetes could now be saved.

Then, the reports of previously unknown complications started to appear. Although insulin significantly prolonged the lives of diabetics, it had by no means cured diabetes. For some reason that was very difficult to identify, many people who had insulin-dependent diabetes for ten or more years began to develop long-term complications. The question was, why?

It became increasingly clear that, although insulin was lifesaving for people with IDDM, its use did not guarantee normal blood sugar control. In fact, because this was before self-monitoring, before the different types of insulin were available, and before the concept of coordinating insulin, diet, and exercise, normal glucose control was not possible. Nevertheless, even thirty years ago, many physicians began to espouse tight control as a means of preventing long-term complications. Other physicians, noting that there was no proof that attempts to control blood sugar improved long-term outcome, did not recommend intensive therapy.

The main point of debate was whether chronic high blood sugar levels were themselves the cause of complications. There were several competing theories, some of which were quite credible: by-products of carbohydrate metabolism, autoimmune processes, or some other effect of IDDM independent of blood glucose control could have been the culprit. In any case, there was no way to examine the impact of tight control on complications, because the methods for measuring blood sugar and complications were crude, and there was no realistic way for patients to achieve glucose control in the near-normal range.

Then, in the late 1970s, new self-testing methods for blood sugar were developed. Almost overnight, it became possible for people with diabetes to check their blood sugar almost anywhere and anytime, with accuracy that had never before been available in self-testing. People with diabetes could find out their precise blood sugar *at that moment,* instead of guessing it on the basis of a urine test. With rapid, accurate glucose measurement available, new therapies that could achieve and maintain near-normal glucose levels were developed. Finally, the hemoglobin A1c assay provided an objective means of measuring long-term metabolic control, and other research methods were developed to measure eye, kidney, and nerve disease.

The opportunity to test whether intensive therapy would improve the long-term prospects of people with diabetes was finally at hand. If people with diabetes could improve their blood sugar control—not so that it was *perfect,* mind you, because perfect control is almost impossible for someone without a functioning pancreas—then it would be possible to test the effect that improved blood sugar control had on complications. Thus was born the DCCT. Diabetes researchers from all over the United States and Canada teamed up to design the study and then find willing patients and talented coworkers with the time and dedication to participate in a ten-year experiment.

The task of administering the DCCT was daunting. Twenty-nine medical institutions, including Mass General, cooperated in recruiting, selecting, training, and then, of course, following patients.

Fifty-six patients at Mass General joined the study. All 1,441 patients involved in the study had had IDDM for at least one year, and not longer than fifteen years. To be eligible, volunteers had to be between thirteen and thirty-nine years of age, and they had to be taking no more than two injections of insulin a day prior to joining the study. At the start of the study, approximately one half of the patients had no signs of complications; the other half had mild-to-moderate retinopathy. The group was split evenly between female and male volunteers.

The Study Design

Any research study, to be effective, must be devised to answer specific questions. The DCCT was designed to answer two separate but related questions:

• Will intensive therapy aimed at achieving glucose control as close to the normal range as possible prevent the development of long-term complications in IDDM patients who have no evidence of complications at the start of the study?
• Will intensive therapy affect the progression of complications in IDDM patients who have at least minimal complications?

Once we had recruited the patients, they were randomly assigned to one of two treatment groups. The randomization process, as it is called, ensured that no bias—unintended or otherwise—would arise in the way patients were assigned to the two treatments. Randomization makes the results of the study more reliable.

The first treatment group was the "experimental," or intensive treatment group; they were treated with the intervention we hoped would decrease the occurrence and progression of complications. Intensive therapy included a demanding regimen of diabetes control composed of at least three doses of insulin per day, given either by injection or with an insulin pump (see Chapter 5). Intensive therapy required monitoring of blood sugar levels at least four times a day in order to adjust insulin doses appropriately, and once a week at 3 A.M., just to make sure that overnight blood sugar levels were kept in a safe range. Intensive therapy patients were taught to adjust their insulin dosage to account for day-to-day changes in their food intake and exercise level. The day-to-day goal was to keep pre-meal blood sugars between 70 and 120 mg/dl and the peak blood sugar after meals less than 180 mg/dl. Our overall goal for the intensive therapy group was to lower their hemoglobin A1c levels—a measure of the average level of glucose control over the previous two to three months—into the normal range (see Chapter 3).

In addition to the participants' responsibilities for frequent injections and monitoring, and careful attention to diet, exercise, and all the other factors that might affect sugar control, intensive therapy required intensive education and frequent follow-up by the management team, including nurse educators, dietitians, and physicians.

The second treatment group was the "control" group. Such a group is a necessary component of any clinical trial; members of this group provide a basis for comparison for the results in the experimental treatment group. The control group followed conventional therapy: no more than two shots of insulin per day, and daily monitoring. The goal of treatment in the conventional therapy group was to maintain normal growth and development and to prevent symptoms of either hyper- or hypoglycemia. However, patients were not given specific hemoglobin A1c or blood sugar goals.

What the DCCT Showed

Everyone enrolled in the study was periodically tested to monitor the onset or progression of complications, including retinopathy (eye), nephropathy (kidney), and neuropathy (nervous system). The average patient was followed for six-and-a-half years, with a range of four to more than nine years.

Although intensive therapy was very effective in lowering glucose and hemoglobin A1c levels, most of the patients in the intensive therapy group had trouble keeping their hemoglobin A1c in the normal range. Over the course of the study, average hemoglobin A1c in the intensive therapy group was approximately 7 percent, or 2 percent lower than with conventional therapy. Average blood sugar levels were about 70 to 80 mg/dl lower. The impact of keeping blood sugar levels just this much closer to normal was starkly illustrated in the clinical outcomes of the study. In fact, the results of the study were so conclusive that it was stopped one year earlier than we had planned, just so we could get this information to the public as quickly as possible. Let's learn about the results now.

Eye Disease

Although we looked at the effect of intensive treatment on all the major complications of diabetes, diabetic eye disease was the primary focus of our attention. For the first three years, there was little difference between the two groups in the development or progression of retinopathy, as measured by the eye photographs we took. However, from that point on, it was apparent that considerably more retinal damage was taking place in the conventional treatment group, while the intensive therapy group remained relatively stable. Five years into the study, there were twice as many people with retinopathy among those receiving conventional treatment than among those getting intensive treatment. As the study went on, we could see that there was a dramatic difference between the two groups; by the time we had followed patients for six years, ninety-one conventionally treated patients had retinopathy, whereas only twenty-three intensively treated patients did. Overall, intensive therapy reduced the risk of developing clinical eye disease by *76 percent*. We also noticed that, among people who had mild to moderate retinopathy at the beginning of the study, intensive treatment reduced its progression by more than 50 percent. Finally, intensive therapy reduced the development of severe eye disease and the need for laser treatment by about 50 percent. Thus, intensive treatment was highly effective at improving long-term eye disease at all of the stages studied in the DCCT. It both prevented the development of and slowed the progression of diabetic retinopathy.

Kidney Disease

The development of kidney disease is a slow, insidious process that can take as long as twenty-five years. The study itself only lasted ten years, so it wasn't practical to wait and see which study participants went on to develop kidney failure.

This doesn't mean the study offered no guidance on the effect of intensive therapy on the progression of kidney disease, however. Several early signs or predictors of diabetic kidney disease have been identified whose presence indicates that severe kidney disease is much more likely to develop. Preventing the development of, or decreasing, these predictors is likely to reduce the chance that severe kidney disease will develop. To detect kidney disease as early as possible, we normally test for increased excretion, or leakage, of albumin into the urine. Albumin is a protein found in very high quantities in the blood. Normally, only small amounts of albumin are filtered into the urine, and most of it is reabsorbed, with the result that very small amounts (usually less than 20 mg per day) appear in the urine. With early kidney abnormalities in diabetes, increasing amounts of albumin appear in the urine—usually more than 30 to 40 mg daily, known as microalbuminuria. As kidney disease progresses, the urine levels rise into the thousands of milligrams per day. When albumin excretion increases beyond 300 mg per day, it is no longer called microalbuminuria, but is termed *albuminuria* or *clinical grade albuminuria*.

In the DCCT, we examined the effect of intensive treatment on the level of albumin excretion. Again, the results were impressive. People on intensive therapy were one third less likely to develop elevated microalbuminuria than the conventional therapy group. The intensive therapy group also had about half the risk (56 percent lower) of developing clinical grade albuminuria than the conventional therapy group. Because so few patients in the study actually developed advanced kidney disease, for the reasons discussed above, we can't look at differences between the two groups as statistically valid. Nevertheless, only two people on intensive treatment developed advanced kidney disease, compared with five in the conventional treatment group.

Neuropathy

As we've seen in Chapter 9, peripheral neuropathy can be either painful or painless, or it can cause numbness. For the purposes of the study, we also included in our definition of neuropathy the appearance of abnormalities in nerve conduction tests. Five years into the study, we looked at patients who had entered the study without any signs of neuropathy. Ten percent of these people who had been treated with conventional therapy demonstrated signs of neuropathy, whereas only 3 percent of the intensive therapy patients did. Intensive therapy reduced the development of neuropathy by 60 percent.

Heart Disease

Because the people in the study were relatively young (thirteen to thirty-nine years), we knew that it was unlikely that we would see significant numbers of cases of heart disease. However, we were able to look at one of the main predisposing factors for heart disease, low-density lipoprotein cholesterol, or LDL cholesterol as it is better known. A level of LDL cholesterol higher than 160 mg/dl is generally considered a risk factor for heart disease. We found that intensive therapy reduced the development of high LDL cholesterol levels by 34 percent.

Hypoglycemia and Other Adverse Effects

If there is any overall disadvantage to tight blood sugar control, it is that it puts patients at higher risk for hypoglycemia, often called an insulin reaction. The symptoms of hypoglycemia occur when blood sugar drops to a point where cells in the brain receive inadequate nutrition (see Chapter 7). It's often accompanied by the physical symptoms of sweatiness, shaking, and mental confusion. If not treated, severe hypoglycemia can result in coma and, rarely, even death. For people with diabetes, it's important to be able to recognize the signs of hypoglycemia, and to know how to treat it properly. It is also a good backup for spouses and other close acquaintances to be familiar with the signs in case of an emergency.

People with diabetes who have been able to lower their blood sugars to close to the normal range often find that they are more likely to dip into the hypoglycemic range from time to time. This is exactly what happened to the participants in the DCCT: hypoglycemia was three times as common in the intensive therapy group than in the conventional therapy group. Hypoglycemia resulting in coma or seizure was relatively rare compared to the overall number of "insulin reactions"; still, they occurred three times more often in people undergoing intensive therapy. What's important to remember is that no deaths or disabilities in either group were attributable to hypoglycemia. Over the nine years of the study (almost 10,000 "patient-years"), there were fifty-four incidents in which patients in the intensive therapy group were hospitalized for hypoglycemia, compared to thirty-six in the conventional therapy group. The good news is that almost all of these hospitalizations were brief and uncomplicated.

If you look at this as a choice between evils—the short-term problems of hypoglycemia that accompany tight blood sugar control, versus the long-term complications associated with chronic high blood sugar—you should have no difficulty at all seeing which is the lesser of the two. The DCCT Research Group concluded that, although intensive therapy needed to be implemented carefully to minimize hypoglycemia, it was clearly the best choice of therapy for most people with IDDM. Choosing to keep your blood sugar under tight control is a wise long-term investment: there may be some bumpy spots along the way, but several years down the road, it will pay off with better health.

Non-Insulin-Dependent Diabetes Mellitus and the DCCT

There are many differences between IDDM (type I diabetes) and NIDDM (type II diabetes). However, they do share some major features: they both involve failure of the body to control blood sugar adequately, and both leave patients vulnerable to significant complications such as the ones discussed above.

The DCCT showed that intensive therapy can help people with IDDM avoid complications. However, the DCCT looked only at patients with IDDM; no one with NIDDM was involved. Consequently, the question remains: What significance does the DCCT have for people with NIDDM? Is intensive therapy with tight blood sugar control appropriate for them, or not? The American

Diabetes Association stated that "it seems reasonable to recommend tight control in many patients with non-insulin-dependent disease. . . ." Considering that intensive therapy is so highly recommended in diabetics with IDDM, this somewhat fainter praise suggests that the medical community has not come to a firm decision.

It's clear that tight blood sugar control has advantages for people with IDDM, and will probably benefit people with NIDDM. As pointed out earlier, many people with NIDDM can potentially achieve tight blood sugar control through diet and exercise, without even using insulin or oral agents.

However, I think we must acknowledge that the jury is still out as to whether all people with NIDDM should aim to control their blood sugar at all costs. The main reason for our indecision is that the therapy to achieve near-normal glucose levels for people with NIDDM can be quite different from the therapy we prescribe for people with IDDM. These NIDDM therapies have not been directly studied in long-term trials. Thus, it is difficult to weigh the long-term benefits against the risks, as was done in the DCCT. Tight blood sugar control in some people with NIDDM necessitates very high doses of insulin (see Chapter 10), which could result in even greater weight gain. We don't know whether the benefit of lower sugars balances the risk of weight gain. These important differences between the two populations make it impossible to say that intensive therapy with tight blood sugar control is appropriate for everybody with NIDDM.

Is Intensive Treatment for Everyone?

Whether or not elevated blood sugar levels actually *cause* complications, it's clear from our study that *controlling* blood sugar reduces the long-term complications of diabetes. However, the adverse effects of therapy, and hypoglycemia in particular, have to be taken into account. Despite the impressive results of the DCCT, there are certainly some people for whom intensive therapy may not be appropriate.

To begin with, there are some people with IDDM who, for various reasons, might not benefit from intensive treatment. For example, a small proportion of people with long-term IDDM have blood sugar levels that fluctuate widely, yet these people have managed to avoid complications despite having had diabetes for years. There are clearly some protective mechanisms operating in these people that we just haven't yet identified, and it makes no sense to alter their self-treatment plan if it's working for them, psychologically and physically. Many elderly people are also frail, and vulnerable to all sorts of sprains, breaks, and fractures. It's probably risky to put an elderly, frail person in a position where hypoglycemia might cause a fall and a broken hip or shoulder.

There are also people whose complications are so far advanced that intensive treatment will serve only to complicate their treatment plan even further. In people whose kidneys are failing, for instance, it's unlikely that tight blood sugar control will provide them with any additional benefit.

People who make their living in dangerous occupations might also be poor candidates for intensive therapy. I've always maintained that anyone who's operating a crane with a wrecking ball outside of your office building ought to have a blood sugar safely above 150, just to make sure that he or she has a steady hand. It's important to use common sense when trying to regulate blood sugar closely in people who might easily injure themselves or others.

Also, not everyone will have access to the kind of treatment team we think is necessary for intensive treatment. It's not clear that family practitioners or general practitioners, who have traditionally provided a high proportion of diabetes care to people with both IDDM and NIDDM, have either the time or the expertise to deal with the demands of intensive treatment.

Many people with diabetes will be disappointed to learn that intensive treatment comes at additional financial cost. The increased attention from diabetologist, diabetic nurse educator, and dietitian all cost more. Intensive treatment may also require you to spend more on diabetes supplies: insulin, syringes, alcohol wipes. If you're injecting insulin only twice a day now, costs for these supplies are likely to double, and perhaps rise even more. There are additional costs involved in switching to a pump (see Chapter 5).

Intensive treatment involves setting some very hard-to-achieve goals and sticking to them. It isn't realistic to think that everyone will be able to reach those goals, but if most people are able to improve their blood sugar even if only by 20 to 40 points, it may allow them to avoid complications for several years and decrease the rate of progression if those complications occur. This may be one of the most important lessons from the DCCT—lower is better, assuming that you can avoid hypoglycemia.

There's no law that says we have to do exactly what our doctors, nurse educators, and dietitians tell us to do. What the DCCT offers us is a therapy that has been carefully studied and proven to result in better health. Keeping blood sugars as close as possible to the normal range will help prevent the complications of diabetes. I think it's important to stress again that this is not the opinion of the "four out of five doctors" we hear about so often in the media. This was a large-scale experiment that was carried out in the nation's most prestigious hospitals under rigorous scientific conditions. Consider it, and make your choice.

The results of the DCCT provide the means of preventing and slowing the progression of diabetic complications that are responsible for much of the suffering that accompanies diabetes. We now have a blueprint for the future of diabetes care.

Index

acarbose (Precose), 144, 250–51
ACE inhibitors, 166, 194–95
acidosis, 57, 249
adrenaline, 132
adult onset diabetes, 15–16
aging, and NIDDM, 5
albumin, 161, 163
albuminuria, 161, 165, 166, 264–65
Allen diet, 57
aloneness, 7, 24, 36–37
American Diabetic Association (ADA), nutritional guidelines from, 65, 79, 236–37
amniocentesis, 217
amputations, 182, 184, 197
anemia, 162, 165
angina, 183, 187
angiography, fluorescein, 154
angioplasty, 196–97
animal species insulin, 97
APGAR scale, 219
aspartame, 70–71
atherosclerosis, 181
autoimmune diseases, 16
autonomic neuropathy, 174

babies:
    APGAR scale for, 219
    and birth trauma, 216–17
    birth weight of, 215, 217–18, 223
    breastfeeding, 220–21
    due date of, 215–16
    and failing labor, 218
    and hypoglycemia, 220, 223
    induced delivery of, 216
    lungs of, 215, 216, 217–18, 219, 223
    in NICU, 219–20
    pancreas of, 220
    and shoulder dystocia, 215, 217
    size of, 215, 216, 217
    see also fetus
balloon angioplasty, 196–97
behavioralists, 53–54
behaviors, 7–8
beta-adrenergic blockers, 195
beta cells:
    destruction of, 16, 17–18, 20, 112
    and pregnancy, 220, 224
bile acid sequestrants, 192
birth defects, 209–10, 211
birth trauma, 216–17
birth weight, 215, 217–18, 223
bladder problems, 178
blaming the patient, 8
blood:
    acidity of, 18, 57
    proteins in, 165
blood lipids, 53, 193, 225
blood pressure:
    and exercise, 243
    high, see high blood pressure
    low, 178–79

blood sugar, 9
  and complications, 147, 259, 269
  and DCCT, *see* Diabetes Control and Complications Trial
  and diet, *see* diet
  and eating habits, 60–61
  and exercise, 115, 118, 120–21, 242–43, 244
  and GDM, 23, 223
  glucose tolerance test of, 28–29, 223
  glucose transporters, 84
  and hormones, 86
  and hypoglycemia, *see* hypoglycemia
  and IDDM, 18–20
  and insulin, 18, 20, 57, 83–90, 118, 239
  measurements of, 9, 28–29
  and medications, 256
  monitors of, 13, 57–58, 89–90
  and NIDDM, 20–21, 111, 230, 239, 242, 246
  and obesity, 231–32
  and pregnancy, 208–9, 211–14, 219–20
  self-monitoring of, 58, 88–90, 143, 214, 259
  sensors of, 13
  steady levels of, 19–20
  and sugar substitutes, 71
  tight control of, 11–14, 39, 59–60, 147–49, 176–77, 258–59, 266–67, 268, 269–71
  and triglycerides, 193–94
  and weight control, 21, 227
blood vessels, *see* macrovascular disease
bolus, 105
bone thinning, 162
brain, blood supply to, 184–85
breastfeeding, 220–21

CABG (coronary artery bypass graft), 188, 196
calcium channel blockers, 195
calluses and corns, 201–2
calorie counting, 234–37
carbohydrates:
  counting, 74, 80–82
  liquid, 233
  oral, 140–42, 214
cardiologists, 53, 188
cardiovascular disease, 11
  and exercise, 116, 241
  and weight, 65
  see also heart disease; macrovascular disease
carotid arteries, 182, 184
carotid endarterectomy, 197
carpal tunnel syndrome, 177
cataracts, diabetic, 157
catheters, 104–5, 188
cesarean section, 218, 223
Charcot foot, 202
children:
  caregivers of, 135
  hypoglycemia in, 134–35
  and juvenile diabetes, 15–16
  and retinopathy, 151
cholesterol, 53
  and exercise, 241
  and heart disease, 190–92, 238–39, 265–66
  and kidney failure, 181
  and NIDDM, 225, 238–39, 241
cholesterol-lowering drugs, 192–94
circulation, 53
  and amputations, 182, 184
  collateral, 197
  and exercise, 116, 241
  and healing, 11
  and peripheral vascular disease, 181–85, 188, 197
clear insulin, 93–94
clinical grade albuminuria, 264
complications, 6, 145–203
  and blood sugar, 147, 259, 269

classes of, 149–50
and DCCT, 11–14, 258, 260, 262
and diet, 57, 88
eye disease, 150–59
foot problems, 197–203
and GDM, 23, 147
and high blood pressure, 149
kidney disease, 159–71
macrovascular disease, 150, 179–97
and metabolism, 146–47
and microvasculature, 147
neuropathy, 171–79
and NIDDM, 20
and self-care, 145–46, 149
and specialists, 52–54
and tight blood sugar control, 11, 39, 147–49, 258–59, 269–71
and undertreatment, 13
concealment, 7
congenital malformations, 209–10
corns and calluses, 201–2
coronary arteries, 196
coronary artery bypass graft (CABG), 188, 196
cotton wool spot, in eye, 152
creatinine, 165, 170
cultural conditions, 5, 56, 227

DCCT, see Diabetes Control and Complications Trial
dehydration, 18, 57, 118
denial, 22, 29, 33
diabetes:
    central problem of, 9
    complications of, see complications
    costs of, 6–7
    diagnosis of, see diagnosis
    drug-induced, 23
    and genetic syndromes, 23
    history of, 8–10, 258
    as inherited, 221–22
    meaning of term, 8
    and pancreatic diseases, 23
    and philosophical changes, 14–15
    research on, 254–55; see also Diabetes Control and Complications Trial
    symptoms of, 16–17, 18, 26–27
    see also IDDM, NIDDM
Diabetes Control and Complications Trial (DCCT), 11–12, 14, 254–71
    control group in, 261–62
    and diagnosis, 32–33
    and diet, 59–60, 61
    experimental group in, 261
    findings of, 262–67
    and hypoglycemia, 133–34, 266–67
    and IDDM, 256
    and MDI, 98–104
    and NIDDM, 267–68
    patient cooperation in, 257–58
    purposes of, 258–60
    study design for, 260–62
    and tight blood sugar control, 59–60, 147–49, 266–67, 268, 269–71
Diabetes Forecast (ADA), 236
diabetes mellitus, meaning of term, 8–9
Diabetes Self-Management (ADA), 236
diabetologists, 27–28, 39–45
    flow charts of, 42–43
    functions of, 40–41
    and NIDDM, 213
diagnosis, 3–4, 6, 25–37
    acceptance of, 31–33, 35–37
    blood sugar measurement, 28–29
    and DCCT, 32–33
    and denial, 22, 29, 33
    and family members, 33–34
    and honeymoon phase, 29–30
    and lifestyle, 31–33, 34–35
    and positive attitude, 35
    symptoms and, 26–27

dialysis, 166–67
diet, 31, 55–82
    ADA guidelines for, 65, 79,
        236–37
    Allen, 57
    and blood sugar, 57, 59–61,
        238
    breaking, 238–39
    calorie counting, 234–37
    carbohydrate counting, 74,
        80–82
    and culture, 56
    and DCCT, 59–60, 61
    diary of, 47–48, 231
    and dietitian, 50–52, 231
    and eating habits, 60–61, 227,
        231–39
    exchange system in, 58–59,
        74, 78–80
    fat in, 65–66, 72, 237, 238–39
    fiber in, 67, 178
    and food labels, 71, 72
    of food robots, 43
    general nutritional guidelines,
        65–74
    Healthy Food Choices, 73,
        75–78
    and heart disease, 190–94,
        238–39
    and the human factor, 56–57,
        63–64
    individual guidelines of, 73,
        74
    and insulin, 57–58
    liquid carbohydrates in,
        233
    meal planning in, 65, 73–74
    moderation in, 47
    and NIDDM, 226–40
    salt in, 67, 179, 190
    sample menus, 73
    sugar in, 67–71, 73–74
    traditional vs. modern
        approach to, 62–64
    vegetarian, 66
dietitian, 50–52, 231
dilated-eye examinations, 153–54
diuretics, 194

DKA (diabetic ketoacidosis),
        18–19, 91–92, 226, 243
drug-induced diabetes, 23

eating, frequent, 28
eating habits:
    and blood sugar, 60–61
    and NIDDM, 227, 231–39
edema:
    and kidneys, 161–62, 163
    macular, 152, 154, 155
endocrinologists, 27–28, 39–45
entrapment syndromes, 177–78
environmental conditions, 5
Exchange Lists for Meal Planning
        (ADA), 79
exchange system, 58–59, 74,
        78–80
exercise, 114–28
    benefits of, 240–43
    and blood sugar, 115, 118,
        120–21, 242–43, 244
    with a buddy, 124
    cautions about, 118–19, 128,
        243–44
    and circulation, 116, 241
    and dehydration, 118
    do's and don'ts of, 128
    and eye problems, 119, 244
    and foot problems, 119, 244
    goals of, 127–28
    and heart disease, 116–17,
        190, 241
    and heart rate, 121–22, 124
    and IDAA, 124–26
    and IDDM, 116, 118
    and injection sites, 123
    and insulin, 118, 241
    and ketones, 118
    low-impact, 245
    and metabolism, 116, 228–29,
        241
    and neuropathy, 118, 243–44
    and NIDDM, 116, 228–30,
        240–45
    physical exam before, 244
    with portable step, 124
    protective effect of, 240

side effects of, 243–44
and Theraband, 123
walking, 117, 245
and weight loss, 116, 228–30
exercise tolerance test, 187
exudates, 152
eyes:
    cataracts in, 157
    double vision, 173
    examinations of, 153–54
    and exercise, 119, 244
    floaters in, 156
    laser treatment of, 149, 155
    and legal blindness, 157–58
    macula of, 152
    night vision, 155
    and ophthalmologists, 52
    physical operation of, 150
    visual field of, 155
    see also retinopathy

family members:
    and diagnosis, 33–34
    frustration of, 45
    and hypoglycemia, 138–40
    injections by, 101–2
    parents, 44, 49
fat:
    in diet, 65–66, 72, 237,
        238–39
    as energy source, 84
fat cells:
    and blood sugar, 18
    and insulin, 57, 85–87
fetus:
    activity of, 219
    and birth defects, 209–10, 211
    development of, 210–13, 215,
        217–18
fiber, in diet, 67, 178
fibric acids, 194
fitness, see exercise
fluid intake, 18
fluorescein angiography, 154
focal neuropathy, 173–74, 177
folate, 211
food, see diet
foot care, 53, 197–203

and amputations, 197
calluses and corns, 201–2
and Charcot foot, 202
and complications, 149, 150,
    198–99
and dry skin, 200–201
and exercise, 119, 244
and footwear, 201
heels, 200–201
and insensitive feet, 199
inspection, 200
and symptoms, 202
toenails, 201
and ulceration, 173, 183–84,
    201
washing, 199–200
foot drop, 173
friends, and hypoglycemia,
    138–40
fructose, 71

gastroparesis, 174–76, 178
GDM (gestational diabetes
    mellitus), 22–23, 222–24
    and complications, 23, 147
    guidelines for care of, 209
    and NIDDM, 22, 207
    screening for, 223
gemfibrozil, 194
genetic syndromes, 23
glomeruli, 160
glucagon, 140–42, 214
Glucophage (metformin), 144,
    224, 248–50
glucose, see blood sugar

hands:
    carpal tunnel syndrome, 177
    and neuropathy, 171
health care costs, 6–7
Healthy Food Choices, 73, 75–78
heart attack, see myocardial
    infarction (MI)
heart disease, 11, 53, 180–97
    atherosclerosis, 181
    DCCT findings on, 265–66
    diagnosis of, 185–89
    and diet, 190–94, 238–39

heart disease (cont'd)
  and exercise, 116–17, 190, 241
  heart attack, 181, 187
  and NIDDM, 226, 238–39
  risk factors for, 180–81, 185–86, 189–90
  and surgery, 196–97
  treatment of, 189–95
heart rate:
  and pulse, 121
  resting, 121, 174
  target, 121–22, 124
hemodialysis, 166–67
hemoglobin A1c assay, 259
hemorrhages, in retina, 151–52
high blood pressure, 53
  and complications, 149
  and diet, 190
  and drugs, 194–95
  effects of, 180
  and kidney disease, 162–63, 165–66
  and NIDDM, 225, 243
high blood sugar, see hyperglycemia
HLA match, 170
HMG-CoA reductase inhibitors, 193
honeymoon phase, 29–30, 110
hormones:
  counter-regulatory, 86
  and insulin, 83, 214
Humalog, 94
human factor, and diet, 56–57, 63–64
human recombinant insulin, 97
hyperglycemia, 21
hyperlipidemia, 193
hypertension, 149, 194
  see also high blood pressure
hypoglycemia, 129–44
  and adrenaline, 132
  babies and, 220, 223
  cause of, 131, 266
  in children, 134–35
  and DCCT, 133–34, 266–67

family and friends and, 138–40
and glucagon, 140–42, 214
and IDDM, 109, 113, 139
and insulin, 86, 87, 94, 109, 113
in newborn babies, 220, 223
and NIDDM, 113, 143–44
and orthostatic hypotension, 179
and pregnancy, 213–14
and sulfonylureas, 144
symptoms of, 131–33, 135–36, 138
treatment of, 136–38
troubleshooting, 142–43
hypoglycemic medications, 246–53
  acarbose, 250–51
  and blood sugar, 31, 256
  insulin, 251–53
  metformin, 248–50
  sulfonylureas, 247–48

ibuprofen, and kidney disease, 165
IDAA (International Diabetes Athletic Association), 124–26
IDDM, 10, 15–20
  and autoimmune reactions, 16
  and beta cells, 17–18, 20, 112
  and blood sugar levels, 18–20
  and DCCT, 256
  and DKA, 91
  and exercise, 116, 118
  and honeymoon phase, 110
  and hypoglycemia, 109, 113, 139
  and insulin, 16, 17–19, 91, 98–104, 109–12, 113
  and macrovascular disease, 179
  and metabolism, 147
  and single injections, 110–11
  symptoms of, 16–17, 18
implantable pumps, 108–9

impotence, 178
incontinence, 178
injections:
  by family members, 101–2
  MDI, 98–104
  mixed split treatment, 99,
    109–10
  pre-exercise sites for, 123
  procedure of, 101–3
  single, 110–11
  subcutaneous, 92, 103
  timing of, 93
injuries, and exercise, 243–44
insulin, 83–113
  abnormalities in, 23
  action profiles for, 95
  animal species, 97
  and blood sugar, 18, 20, 57,
    83–90, 118, 239
  body's production of, 16, 90,
    91, 222
  clear, 93–94
  and diet, 57–58
  discovery of, 9–10, 19,
    258–59
  and DKA, 91–92
  and exercise, 118, 241
  exogenous sources of, 16
  function of, 83–88
  gene for, 40
  high levels of, 17
  how much and when, 90–92
  Humalog, 94
  human recombinant, 97
  and hypoglycemia, 86, 87, 94,
    109–12, 113
  and IDDM, 16, 17–19, 91,
    98–104, 109–12
  injection of, 92, 101–3,
    110–11
  intermediate, 94–96
  lente, 94–96
  long-acting, 95, 96
  low levels of, 17–18
  MDI, 98–104
  and metabolism, 86
  mixed split treatment, 99,
    109–10

and NIDDM, 20, 21, 91, 92,
  110–13, 230, 239, 251–53
NPH, 94–96, 109–10
and pancreas, 16, 90, 91, 222
physiologic amounts of, 226
and pregnancy, 213, 214–15,
  222
premixed, 96–97
pumps for, see insulin pumps
rapid-acting, 93–94, 95
reactions to, 134, 266
70/30, 96–97
single injection, 110–11
sources of, 97
storage of, 97
treatment plans, 98–111
types of, 92–97
ultralente, 96
and weight gain, 230
insulin-dependent diabetes
  mellitus, see IDDM
insulin pumps, 13, 91, 99, 104–9
  and bolus, 105
  and catheter, 104–5
  implantable, 108–9
  and pregnancy, 214–15
insulin resistance, 20, 225–26
International Diabetes Athletic
  Association (IDAA),
  124–26
islet cells, 14, 227
isolation, 7, 24, 36–37

juvenile diabetes, 15–16

ketoacidosis (DKA), 18–19,
  91–92, 226, 243
ketones, 18–19, 118
kidney disease, 11, 53, 150,
  159–71
  DCCT findings on, 264–65
  diagnosis of, 163–65
  and dialysis, 166–67
  end-stage renal failure, 159,
    163, 166
  and heart disease, 181
  and high blood pressure,
    162–63, 165–66

kidney disease (*cont'd*)
symptoms of, 162–63
treatment of, 165–71
kidneys:
and edema, 161–62, 163
functions of, 159–60
glomeruli of, 160
and metformin, 249
scarring of, 162
transplants of, 167–71

lactic acidosis, 249
lente insulin, 94–96
lifestyle:
and causes of diabetes, 5–6
and diagnosis, 31–33, 34–35
diet, 43–44
liver:
and glucagon, 141
and glucose uptake, 84–87
long-acting insulin, 95, 96
lovastatin, 193
low blood pressure, 178–79
low blood sugar, *see*
hypoglycemia
lungs, of babies, 215, 216,
217–18, 219, 223
lymphoma, 169

macrovascular disease, 150,
179–97
and amputation, 182
angina, 183, 187
and circulation, 181–85
intermittent claudication, 183
peripheral, 181–85, 188, 197
see also heart disease
macula, 152
macular edema, 152, 154, 155
magnetic resonance imaging
(MRI), 189
mannitol, 68
MDI (multiple daily injections),
98–104
meal planning, 65, 73–74
calorie counting, 236–37
carbohydrate counting, 74,
80–82

exchange system, 58–59, 74,
78–80
Healthy Food Choices, 73,
75–78
"Month of Meals," 238
see also diet
*Meal-Planning Approaches for
Diabetes Management*
(ADA), 65, 236–37
Medicalert bracelet, 119
medications, 245–53
acarbose, 250–51
and blood sugar, 31, 256
insulin, 251–53
metformin, 248–50
sulfonylureas, 247–48
mellitus, meaning of term, 8
metabolic rate, 232
metabolism, 6
and complications, 146–47
and exercise, 116, 228–29,
241
regulation of, 86
and weight loss, 228–29, 241
metformin (Glucophage), 144,
224, 258–50
MI (myocardial infarction), 181,
187
microalbuminuria, 161, 165,
166, 264–65
microaneurysms, 151–52
microvasculature, 147, 179
"Month of Meals," 238
motivation, 48
motor neuropathy, 171, 177–78
MRI (magnetic resonance
imaging), 189
multiple daily injections (MDI),
98–104
muscles:
and blood sugar, 18
and exercise, 123
and insulin, 57, 85–87
myocardial infarction (MI), 181,
187

nephrologists, 163
nephromegaly, 160

nephropathy, *see* kidney disease
nerve conduction studies, 175
neural tube defects, 210, 211
neuropathy, 53, 147, 150,
    171–79
  autonomic, 174
  and blood sugar control,
    176–77
  DCCT findings on, 265
  diagnosis, 175–76
  and entrapment syndromes,
    177–78
  and exercise, 118, 243–44
  focal, 173–74, 177
  motor, 171, 177–78
  nerves affected by, 171
  peripheral, 202, 265
  sensory, 171, 172, 173, 177,
    183
  symptoms of, 171–75
  treatments for, 177–79
Neutral Protamine Hagedorn
    (NPH) insulin, 94–96,
    109–10
niacin (nicotinic acid), 192–93
NICU, babies in, 219–20
NIDDM, 16, 20–22, 225–53
  and aging, 5
  and blood lipid levels, 225
  and blood sugar, 20–21, 111,
    230, 239, 242, 246
  and calorie counting, 234–37
  and DCCT, 267–68
  and diet, 226–40
  and DKA, 92, 226, 243
  and eating habits, 227,
    231–38
  and exercise, 116, 228–30,
    240–45
  and GDM, 22, 207
  and heart disease, 226,
    238–39
  and high blood pressure, 225,
    243
  and hypoglycemia, 113,
    143–44
  and insulin, 20, 21, 91, 92,
    110–13, 230, 239, 251–53

and insulin resistance, 20,
    225–26
  and insulin secretions, 21
  and macrovascular disease,
    179
  and meal planning, 236–38
  and medications, 245–53
  and metabolism, 147, 228–29,
    241
  in minority groups, 207
  and obesity, 20, 116, 225,
    226–28
  and oral agents, 22
  and single injections, 110–11
  and weight loss, 227–32,
    238–39, 241
non-insulin-dependent diabetes
    mellitus, *see* NIDDM
NPH (Neutral Protamine
    Hagedorn) insulin, 94–96,
    109–10
NSAIDs (nonsteroidal anti-
    inflammatory drugs), 165
nurse educators, 45–50
  and pregnancy, 213
  and self-treatment, 47–48
NutraSweet, 70–71
nutrition, *see* diet

obesity, 6
  and blood sugar, 231–32
  and NIDDM, 20, 116, 225,
    226–28
obstetrics, high-risk, 210–13, 218
One Touch II, 89
ophthalmologists, 52
ophthalmoscope, 153
opium, tincture of, 178
oral agents, 22
oral carbohydrates, 140–42, 214
oral glucose tolerance test, 28–29
organ transplants, 14, 167–71
orthostatic hypotension, 178–79
osteoporosis, 162

pancreas:
  of animals, 97
  of babies, 220

pancreas (*cont'd*)
  diseases of, 23
  and honeymoon phase, 110
  insulin produced in, 16, 90,
    91, 222
  insulin regulated in, 19
  transplants of, 14
parents, 44, 49; *see also* family
  members
peripheral neuropathy, 202,
  265
peripheral vascular disease,
  181–85, 188, 197
peritoneal dialysis, 166
photocoagulation, 155
pitocin, 216
placenta, 222
podiatrists, 53
polydipsia, 18, 27, 28
polyphagis, 28
polyuria, 18, 26, 27, 28
Precose (acarbose), 144, 250–51
pregnancy, 204–24
  and birth defects, 209–10, 211
  and blood sugar control,
    208–9, 211–14, 219–20
  care after delivery, 219–22
  and cesarean section, 218, 223
  and delivery, 215–19
  diabetes care during, 208–19
  of diabetic women, 52, 207,
    208
  and failing labor, 218
  and GDM, 22–23, 207, 209,
    222–24
  and high-risk obstetrics,
    210–13, 218
  and hypoglycemia, 213–14
  and insulin, 213, 214–15, 222
  multidisciplinary team for,
    212–13
  and placenta, 222
protamine, 95
proteins:
  in blood, 165
  in urine, 160–61, 163
psychologists, psychiatrists,
  53–54

radioimmunoassay, 40
rapid-acting insulin, 93–94, 95
regular insulin, 93–94, 109–10
renal failure, 159, 163, 166
research:
  bias in, 261
  clinical trial in, 255
  control group in, 255, 261–62
  and diabetes, 254–55; *see also*
    Diabetes Control and
    Complications Trial
  double-blind trial, 255
  experimental group in, 261
  hemoglobin A1c assay, 259
  patients' roles in, 255
  randomization in, 261
retinopathy, 11, 52, 150–59
  and children, 151
  DCCT findings on, 263
  developmental stages of,
    151–53
  diagnosis of, 153–54
  and exercise, 119
  and IDDM, 151
  and NIDDM, 151
  treatment of, 155–59

saccharin, 70
salt, 67, 179, 190
self-care, 7, 42, 44
  and complications, 145–46,
    149
  consistency in, 47
  control in, 48
  diet diary and, 47–48
  moderation in, 47
  motivation and, 48
self-testing, of blood sugar, 58,
  88–90, 143, 214, 259
sensory neuropathy, 171, 172,
  173, 177, 183
70/30 insulin, 96–97
shoulder dystocia, 215, 217
single injections, 110–11
smoking, 181, 241
sorbitol, 68
split-mixed insulin programs, 99,
  109–10

step, portable, 124
stereoscopic fundus photography, 154
steroids, 169
stress test, 187
strokes, 11, 53, 184–85
sucrose, 69, 71
sugar, 67–71, 73–74
    as energy source, 84
    and hypoglycemia, 136–38
    substitutes for, 68, 70–71
    in urine, 18, 230
    see also blood sugar
sulfonylureas:
    and hypoglycemia, 144
    and NIDDM, 247–48
    and pregnancy, 224
    side effects of, 247–48
    and weight gain, 230

target heart rate, 121–22, 124
technology, 13–14
thallium stress test, 187
Theraband, 123
thirst, 16–17, 18, 27, 28
TIAs (transient ischemic attacks), 184–85
treatment:
    consensus recommendations for, 42
    costs of, 270
    goals of, 270
    intensive, 269–71
treatment team, 38–54, 270
    diabetologist, 39–45
    dietitian, 50–52
    nurse educator, 45–50
    other specialists, 52–54
triglycerides, 193–94
type I diabetes, see IDDM
type II diabetes, see NIDDM

ultralente insulin, 96
ultrasound, 212, 213, 217
undertreatment, 13
University Group Diabetes Program (UGDP), 248
urinary incontinence, 178
urination, frequent, 16–17, 18, 26, 27, 28
urine:
    protein leakage into, 160–61, 163
    sampling of, 164
    sugar in, 18, 230
urine test, 163–64
urologists, 53, 176

vascular surgeons, 53, 202
vegetarian diets, 66

walking, 117, 245
weight, of fetus, 215, 217, 218
weight control:
    and blood sugar, 21, 227
    and cultural conditions, 227
    and eating habits, 231–39
    and exercise, 116, 117, 228–30
    and genetic factors, 227–28
    and ideal weight, 65
    and stress, 228
weight loss, 26–27, 28
    and counting calories, 227
    and metabolism, 228–29, 241
    and NIDDM, 227–32, 238–39, 241
    obstacles to, 227–28

yoga, 245

zinc, and lente insulin, 95

ABOUT THE AUTHORS

DAVID M. NATHAN received his undergraduate education at Amherst College and his medical education and training at the Mt. Sinai School of Medicine in New York and at the Peter Bent Brigham and Massachusetts General Hospitals in Boston, Massachusetts. He has been on the faculty of the Harvard Medical School and the director of the Diabetes Research Center and Diabetes Clinic at the Massachusetts General Hospital for almost twenty years. With more than a hundred publications in the scientific literature, Dr. Nathan is an internationally acknowledged leader in the investigation and care of diabetes and its complications. When he is not tending to athletic injuries (his own), he spends his best hours with his wife Ellen, and his children, Josh and Ben.

JOHN F. LAUERMAN is a freelance writer living in Brookline, Massachusetts. He is a frequent contributor to magazines, newsletters, and books on topics related to health and medicine.